FEAR CANCER NO MORE

Preventive and Healing Information
Everyone Should Know

MAURIS L. EMEKA

Apollo Publishing International

Port Orchard, Washington

Apollo Publishing International
Box 1937
Port Orchard, Washington (98366)

Cover design by Edwina Cusolito.

Publisher's Cataloging in Publication

Emeka, Mauris L.
    Fear cancer no more: preventive and healing
    information everyone should know /
    by Mauris L. Emeka – 1st ed.
    p. cm.
    Includes bibliographical references and index.
ISBN: 0-9640125-6-1

    1. Cancer – Nutritional aspects. 2. Cancer –
Prevention. 3. Cancer – Alternative treatment.
4. Cancer – Popular works. I. Title.

RC268.45.E64 2002   626.99'4
                        QB102-200248

> *For information updates to this book, see*
> **www.cancernomore.com**

DEDICATION

For my beloved Sunday
1943 - 2001

"Each patient carries his own doctor inside him.
They come to us not knowing that truth.
We are at our best when we give the doctor who
resides in each patient a chance to go to work."

Dr. Albert Schweitzer

(The author is donating a portion of the proceeds from the sale of Fear Cancer No More to the Cancer Cure Foundation, a non-profit organization in Newbury Park, California, whose website is: www.cancure.org)

WARNING

The purpose of this book is to add to the growing body of evidence that cancer is an illness caused by nutritional deficiency. I am a researcher and writer, not a physician. The facts presented herein are intended as information only – not as medical advice. I hope that they will provide a basis for readers to make informed decisions. Because there may always be risk involved, even in things that otherwise appear safe and beneficial, the publisher and the author are not responsible for any adverse effects or consequences resulting from the use of any of the suggestions in this book. Please do not read it if you are unwilling to assume that risk. This book encourages the use of health care professionals in connection with cancer therapy; at the same time, it encourages people to take greater responsibility for their own health.

FOREWORD

I awoke June 29, 2001 to the obnoxious ring of an old rotary dial phone. On the other end was my brother with bad news. It was official, Mom had cancer. Six hundred miles away, all I could do was pray. It never entered my mind that in less than four months Mom would depart us.

When my family arrived at my parents' home on the fourth of July everything seemed normal, maybe even better than normal. We celebrated our family's reunion, but something was clearly uneasy about the day. Amidst our recounting of childhood dramas and our laughter there was worry.

I kept telling myself, "she doesn't look sick" and "she'll get through it."

Meanwhile my mother, who had never been one to turn down the finer things in life (i.e., barbequed salmon and homemade ice cream) had to on this night.

For months now, she had found that her body couldn't handle food after about four o'clock in the afternoon. Still, she basked in the warmth of her family – smiling, laughing and just being Mom. My father, was only intermittently involved in the festivities. He seemed to disappear and then reappear every so often. When my curiosity overtook the joy of being in such good company, I ventured back to my father's office where I found him enthralled with something on his computer screen. As I looked closer at the screen I saw the words "pancreas" and "cancer."

Over the course of the following months I found Pop in front of that screen at all hours of the day and night – often with a book in his lap with a title like "One Answer to Cancer" used to cross reference his Internet discoveries as he sought a solution to this our family's most profound problem. This book that you are reading has been my father's greatest distraction, and at the same time his best therapy in the wake of his partner's passing. It is a product of some regret: regret that medical doctors had no solution for Mom's cancer (which they readily admitted) and therefore proceeded to treat rather than cure her as is too often the case with cancer, regret that we did not know then what we know now, regret that the medical establishment seems not to know what our family now knows, regret that the cancer epidemic continues to take the lives of mothers, fathers, brothers and sisters everywhere when its prevention, and even cure, may very well be as close as the local grocery store.

My father has long been interested in diet and health-related issues. This book is the culmination of his crash course on the physiology of cancer. It is important to know that my Pop is not a doctor, though he is a student of cancer's causes and cures. However, with regard to the origin and nature of cancer, many medical practitioners cannot, and often do not, claim to be much more. In any case, we are supremely confident that Mom would have benefited from the information in the following chapters – it might have saved her life had we known it sooner. Cancer has lost much of it's mystery in our family. If we encounter it again, we will know just what to do. In fact, Pop and my wife and child are already doing it. The best way to deal with cancer is not to get it! The intent of this book is to show you how to do that, and if you currently have cancer to point you in the direction for overcoming it. Mom's death was not in vain.

Amon S. Emeka
Port Orchard, Washington
March 31, 2002

ACKNOWLEDGMENTS

This book could not have become a reality without the generous assistance and moral support from a number of people. I am grateful for the manuscript editing, along with words of encouragement from Debra Munn, Vivian Phillips, and Catharine Smith Jones, as well as from family members of the Emeka clan, including Amon, Gabriel, Justin, Apollo, Anjie, Raquel and Farah. I thank my sister Vonnelle Middleton, who first encouraged me to write this book. Finally, a hearty thanks to Ron Snowden of Graphics West (in Seattle) for his work in typesetting the book for final printing, and to Edwina Cusolito for her uniquely creative talent in designing the cover.

Last but not least, I am deeply grateful to Dr. William D. Kelley, whose writing first inspired me to inquire into the root cause of cancer. I truly appreciate Dr. Kelley taking time during our many telephone conversations to explain the nature of cancer, and what each of us as individuals can do about it.

AUTHOR'S NOTE

In July 2001, Sunday Emeka, my dear and loving wife of thirty-six years, was diagnosed with pancreatic cancer. Four months later, and after considerable pain, she made her transition from this life. This heart breaking experience prompted me to look deeply into the nature and cause of cancer to try to discover everyday things that we can all do to prevent as well as overcome this illness. I felt compelled to share my findings in hopes that it will prevent others from experiencing the pain that my family and I endured.

Writing this book has surely brought a measure of healing to me as well as to my family.

Born in 1941 in a rural community in northeast Arkansas, I have long been interested in health issues, although as a layman and writer rather than as a medical professional. My intention is that this book be a resource of important health information, especially about how the body functions at the cellular level to defend against cancer. Hopefully, it will enable each reader to approach the subject of cancer with more understanding and less fear.

One hundred years ago there was very little cancer in the USA and the rest of the Western World.

Now there is an abundance of cancer. It has even become a major industry. What has changed since 1900? Can this be reversed? It is highly unlikely, as long as the focus is merely on "treating cancer. "

"Treating" cancer is not what this book is about. Instead, it calls our attention to a dietary deficiency along with lifestyle changes, all of which offer the best chance for the body to heal itself of this dreaded illness.

Over the last one hundred years we in the Western World have progressively increased our intake of foods that contain omega 6 fatty acids, while decreasing our consumption of foods that contain omega 3 fatty acids – much to the detriment of our overall health. During that same time, we have significantly increased our intake of cereal grains and decreased our consumption of complex carbohydrates that are found in various root plants, legumes, and in fruits and vegetables. In general, our diets have come to include more animal products and refined grain, and fewer foods that contain antioxidants and vital minerals such as calcium. More and more, it is now being acknowledged that this gradual dietary shift has been a major factor in the increased incidence of degenerative diseases, including cancer.

CONTENTS

INTRODUCTION

"My people are destroyed for lack of knowledge."

— HOSEA 4:6

What if you learned that there were steps you could take on your own that might arrest the growth of existing malignant tumors? What if you discovered that there were products that could help you recover from cancer, or-better yet – prevent it altogether? You would probably go to great lengths to seek out these wonder treatments, wouldn't you? No sum of money, no amount of trouble would be too much, if only you could find ways to eliminate cancer, one of the deadliest scourges of humankind. Yet there is no need to search out exotic locales for mysterious herbs, nor do you need to pay exorbitant prices for wonder drugs from the pharmacist. It may come as a surprise, but the best cancer fighters of all are as near as your local grocery store, health food store, farmer's market and (if you have one) your own fruit and vegetable garden.

Information about the link between diet and cancer has been known for a long time. Scientific studies document and validate information about the health-enhancing properties of many common foods. As early as January 1892, an article in Scientific American magazine stated that: "Cancer is more frequent among branches of the human race where carnivorous habits prevail."

This book attempts to reinforce that link between diet and cancer, and to show how eating the right foods is one of the best ways to maintain or restore our health.

During the last one hundred years, Americans in particular and Westerners in general have suffered from cancer at an ever increasing rate. Health professionals and statisticians who follow the numbers tell us that in North America one out of two men, and two out of three women will be diagnosed with the disease at some point during their lives, and the percentage is steadily climbing. Cancer is even striking children at ever younger ages. It used to be that children rarely got cancer. Why? What are we doing differently? Do we have the wisdom and the will power to make some fundamental changes in our living and dietary practices? Or, will we continue hoping (against the odds) for a magic pill to finally emerge from a science lab?

Alarmingly, cancer seems poised to replace heart disease as the number one cause of death in spite of the fact that America declared war on cancer in 1971, and has since spent over $1.5 trillion on conventional cancer research and treatment[1]. Money spent on chemotherapy and radiation has increased at an incredible rate, and so has cancer related deaths.

"In 1990, $3.53 billion was spent on chemotherapy. By 1994 that figure had more than doubled to $7.51 billion. This relentless increase in chemo use was accompanied by a relentless increase in cancer deaths."[2]

Clearly, we are not winning the so called war against cancer, despite the fact that we are continually encouraged to go for frequent check-ups. And the present strategy of devoting billions of dollars to research is at best helping to manage and control cancer, not to eliminate it.

If there is a long range strategy for curing cancer, it is definitely not working. On the other hand, something is working. It is that there are thousands of people (often sincere and well meaning) who profit from a multi-billion dollar cancer industry; they include medical practitioners, cancer fundraising personnel, hospitals, researchers and pharmaceutical companies.

Regrettably, what has emerged over the years since the "war on cancer" is an expensive and profitable industry that does much to control this illness, yet brings us no closer to a cure. The year 2001 saw employment rates drop in the USA, and stock markets fell significantly, but the pharmaceutical industry continued its reign as the most profitable industry in the annual Fortune 500 list. In fact, the ten drug companies in the Fortune 500 topped all three of Fortune magazine's measures of profitability in 2001.

Although it is true that many patients with this illness are now living longer than ever before, the overall death rate continues to rise, and we are faced with a near epidemic. Meanwhile, the billions of dollars spent on cancer research continue to go not as much to identifying the underlying cause of cancer, but to discovering chemical compounds that temporarily check the growth of malignant tumors – and all while cancer continues at an ever increasing pace.

Although it is true that many patients with this illness are now living longer than ever before, the overall death rate continues to rise, and we are faced with a near epidemic. Meanwhile, the billions of dollars spent on cancer research continue to go not as much to identifying the underlying cause of cancer, but to discovering chemical compounds that temporarily check the growth of malignant tumors

– and all while cancer continues at an ever increasing pace.

Too much emphasis is placed on the tumor, and not enough on the cause of the tumor. Surgery, chemotherapy and radiation often shrink the tumor, while at the same time the patient dies from other illnesses brought on by the treatment. Clearly something is wrong here! The tumor itself is not life threatening. But what does endanger the life of the patient is the spreading of cancer throughout the body; and surgery, chemotherapy and radiation do nothing to prevent that.

Considering our lack of success in eradicating this devastating illness, it is no wonder that growing numbers of individuals are pursuing non-traditional approaches to prevent and eliminate cancer on their own.

This is also hardly surprising when we consider that cancer patients are all too often sent home (from the doctor) with few alternatives for treatment outside the narrow set of "conventional" options: surgery, chemotherapy and radiation. However, naturopathic, homeopathic, ayurvedic and other physicians offer a variety of non-toxic treatments that may greatly benefit cancer sufferers. Most importantly however, and the subject of this book, is the self-treatment with healthy foods that complement everything our physicians do for us.

It is time we become aware of something that distinguished scientists proved one hundred years ago: it is that cancer is a chronic metabolic disease arising from dietary deficiency. Cancer is not a germ-related or infectious disease. As such, it is empowering when we come to the understanding that here is an illness we can each influence everyday, depending on our lifestyle choices.

Please do not misunderstand me – I certainly do not recommend that anyone should go it alone in treating any kind of serious illness. But, with a disease such as cancer that affects the body's ability to digest food efficiently and to convert it into energy, the best "physicians" are the patients themselves. They are the ones on the job twenty-four hours a day, who thus have the opportunity to create healthful conditions at the cellular level – conditions that allow the body to successfully interrupt the cycle that otherwise leads to malignant tumor growth.

---

[1] Alternative Medicine & the War on Cancer by Peter Chowka. *Better Nutrition Magazine.* August 1999.

[2] Robert Cathey Research Source. Portland, Oregon. See www.navi.net/~rsc/chemorad.htm

What is Cancer?
How Do We Get It?

We are made victims of sickness, aging, and death by gaps in our knowledge.

– DEEPAK CHOPRA, M.D., AGELESS BODY, TIMELESS MIND

SUMMARY

This chapter explains the underlying causes of cancer as discovered by a distinguished university professor of embryology in Scotland, who researched this topic from 1888 to 1911. Exploring the nature and underlying causes of this illness, this chapter proceeds to discuss what each of us can do about preventing and overcoming it.

Hopefully, this chapter will empower you. It includes the results of scientific research into the underlying cause of cancer. Study it, and you will be in a better position to prevent cancer, or to overcome it.

What is cancer and how does someone get it? According to extensive research in the late nineteenth century by Scottish embryologist Dr. John Beard, the direct cause of cancer is the changing of an ectopic germ cell into an ectopic trophoblast cell in our bodies. By the end of this chapter the reader will understand just what that means.

Admittedly, one of the dangers of writing about the cause of something like cancer is the temptation to oversimplify the situation and offer information that is not adequately supported. That is why I have made a serious effort to carefully study this topic, and I have painstakingly avoided making claims that evidence cannot support. In that regard, this first chapter was the most difficult one to write. It introduces a fundamentally different way of thinking about cancer.

The concepts that describe the root causes of cancer are not easy to explain; and at the outset, the explanations may be challenging for readers. I therefore implore you to approach this chapter with patience, persistence, and an inquisitive mind because many of the concepts offered in the next few pages are the foundation of the remainder of the book. The remaining chapters, except perhaps for chapter eight, represent relatively easy reading. Throughout the book, I have endeavored to write in a conversational style that is not only accurate but accessible to the reader. Having said that, let us now proceed.

HUMAN ENBRYO FORMATION AFFECTS THE POTENTIAL FOR CANCER

In the first week after an egg is fertilized in a woman, the growing mass of cells divides into two kinds, an inner cell mass that embryologists call the embryoblast which becomes the embryo, and an outer layer of cells called the trophoblast which forms the placenta that houses and nourishes the embryo. The embryo goes through various stages of development, and the entire process is so complex that less than half of the developing cell mass ever progresses past the first stage.

As a matter of course, something goes wrong with normal development and many of the cells are actually expelled from the woman's body before they get a chance to implant themselves in the uterus. However, the inner cells that are not expelled manage, along with trophoblast cells, to attach to the wall of the uterus and continue their development. The trophoblast cells then begin rapidly to invade the surrounding tissue, digesting a hole in the wall of the uterus as it makes the placenta. Small blood vessels are disturbed and digested by the invading trophoblast, often forming pools of blood in the tissue that nourishes the growing embryo. While the trophoblast cells aggressively infiltrate surrounding tissue to make the placenta, the inner cell mass of the embryo organizes itself into three primary germ layers (the ectoderm, endoderm and mesoderm), each of which develops into different parts of the human body.

To develop an embryo from these primary germ layers involves precise timing and the extensive migration of various cells from one part of the embryo to another as they proceed with the complex process of forming a human baby. In fact, the timing and orchestration of events within the embryo are nothing short of a miracle. As a result, not every one of these primary germ cells completes a successful development cycle; that means that every human (male and female) contains varying numbers of these primary germ cells that failed to complete their correct migration during the formation of the embryo. These cells are often called "sleeping" or "wandering" cells, and they remain in the developing embryo subsequently circulating throughout the body of the newly formed baby.

These circulating "sleeping" cells are normal in the sense that they are actually in the bodies of all humans and are not a problem until, and unless, they are activated. They can be activated and thus formed into trophoblast cells as a result of a sex hormone imbalance in the body, or as the result of genetic, environmental and nutritional factors. When this happens, it causes a trophoblast (or cancerous) cell mass (similar to the invasive trophoblast cell mass in an expectant mother) to begin forming.

CANCER OCCURS WHEN ECTOPIC GERM CELLS
GIVE WAY TO ECTOPIC TROPHOBLAST CELLS

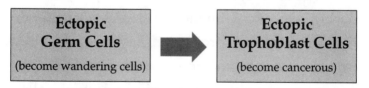

Ordinarily, ectopic germ cells circulate harmlessly in all of us. they are the wandering cells in each of us that did not complete their cycle as part of our early embryonic development. If these wandering cells ever become activated due to various circumstances (like environmental and nutritional factors, or female hormone imbalance) they then give way to ectopic trophoblast cells (or cancer).

This invasive trophoblast cell mass, or spreading tumor, can occur in anyone, and it is what some researchers call a "false placenta" because it is trying to complete a development cycle to form a "baby". I have spoken with pathologists who told me that when cancerous tumors are dissected, it is not uncommon to find within them various types of tissue such as body hair, chips of bones and parts of fingernails, all of which are apparently trying to form into a "baby" – an obvious impossibility, since the misguided (cancerous) cell mass is trying to do the wrong thing at the wrong place and time.

PANCREATIC ENZYMES PREVENT WANDERING CELLS FROM BECOMING CANCEROUS

As previously mentioned, the sleeping or wandering cells circulating in our bodies normally do not cause us any problem. They are prevented from becoming cancerous tumor masses by the presence of circulating protein molecules called enzymes which keep the growth of any activated wandering or sleeping cells in check. These enzymes are generated by the pancreas, and are thus referred to as pancreatic enzymes. Researchers over the years have discovered that cancer cells secrete a protein and starchy coating that covers them and effectively "hides" them from the immune system.

Pancreatic enzymes are extremely important because they can dissolve this coating that covers cancer cells which otherwise enables them to go undetected by the immune system. We can be truly grateful for the work of scientists such as Dr. Beard and others who continued their work; they learned that when our bodies are deficient in certain pancreatic enzymes, the sleeping cells, once they are activated, become cancerous trophoblast cells.

THE ROLE OF THE PANCREAS IS CRUCIAL

The pancreas is an organ in the upper gastrointestinal tract that produces several enzymes. It is commonly known as the organ that makes the enzyme insulin which helps to digest sugar. However, the pancreas also secretes at least four other enzymes critical to the digestion of animal protein, starches (or carbohydrates) and fats. The first two enzymes are trypsin and chymotrypsin which are necessary to digest animal protein. The third is

DIAGRAM OF DIGESTIVE SYSTEM

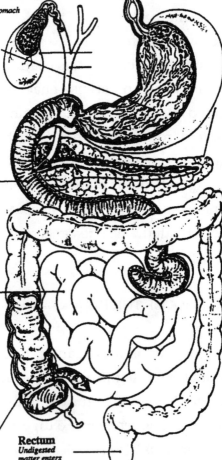

Esophagus
Food is carried down the esophagus by peristaltic action and enters the stomach

Stomach
The pancreatic enzyme must be in an enteric matrix. Food is broken down further by churning and by the action of hydrochloric acid and digestive enzymes secreted by the stomach lining. Food remains in the stomach until it is reduced to a semiliquid consistency (chyme), when it passes into the duodenum.

Duodenum
The pancreatin starts its functions. As food travels along the duodenum, it is broken down further by digestive enzymes from the liver, gallbladder, and pancreas. The duodenum leads directly into the small intestine.

Small Intestine
Additional enzymes secreted by glands in the lining of the small intestine complete the digestive process. Nutrients are absorbed through the intestinal lining into the network of blood vessels and lymph vessels supplying the intestine. Undigested matter passes into the large intestine (the colon).

Colon
Ox Bile is needed to help digest fats. Water in the undigested matter leaving the small intestine is absorbed through the lining of the colon. The residue passes into the rectum.

Pancreas
In some individuals, the pancreas does not produce enough of these enzymes all of the time, therefore supplementation may be a good idea as insurance to assure that there is no deficiency.

Rectum
Undigested matter enters this final part of the large intestine and is expelled.

Anus

This diagram is courtesy of Dr. William D. Kelley

amylase which helps digest starches, and the fourth is lipase which breaks down fats.

Dr. Beard and his successors discovered that these four enzymes, in addition to helping digest our food, are also instrumental in suppressing cancerous trophoblast cells because, as already mentioned, they dissolve the coating that otherwise hides cancer cells and prevents them from being targeted for destruction by the immune system. Therefore, to remain free of cancer, we should always have plenty of these four enzymes circulating in our bodies. These pancreatic enzymes are absolutely essential: they are the sine qua non for cancer resolution.

The pancreas is often greatly challenged as it tries to maintain adequate enzyme production. It should come as no surprise that an early indicator of pancreatic failure (and thus of cancer) is indigestion with belching and passing of excessive gas (flatulence). Persistently foul breath can also be an early indicator, because it signals digestion problems caused by anaerobic bacteria that generate energy without requiring oxygen. As we will see in the next chapter, cancer cells also do not require oxygen. We can help ease the demand placed on the pancreas by substituting harder to digest animal product proteins with easier to digest plant proteins. We would all do well to remember that when the pancreas is overworked, as it often is with the typical Western diet, not only do we risk a shortage of enzymes to digest animal protein, we also risk not having enough of the same enzymes to dissolve the protein and starchy coating from around cancerous cells. Dissolving this coating enables the immune system to finally "see", or recognize, cancer cells and target them for destruction.

When studying the pancreas in detail, one of the first things we learn is that it has a finite capability to produce enzymes. The good news, however, is that all raw foods are loaded with enzymes. In fact, uncooked deep green leafy vegetables have enzyme complexes similar to those produced by the pancreas. The only problem is that most people in the Western world consume a diet of mainly cooked food, and cooking kills the enzymes in the food.

Let us turn our attention again to something that happens in a pregnant woman. At approximately the 56th day of a woman's pregnancy, the growing baby inside the womb develops its own pancreas. When that happens, the baby's pancreatic enzymes (along with the mother's pancreatic enzymes) cause the trophoblast cell mass that forms the placenta (that houses the baby) to stop growing. If the placenta in a pregnant mother continued to grow, it would cause serious problems for both the developing baby and the mother.

Observing the fact that the trophoblast cell mass stopped growing as a result of a certain level of pancreatic enzymes, Dr. John Beard concluded that if people insured that there were sufficient pancreatic enzymes circulating in their bodies, this would stop the growth of otherwise cancerous trophoblast cells.[3]

In other words, if we want to attack cancer at its roots, we must consider ways to introduce more of the appropriate enzymes into our bodies to augment the limited enzyme producing potential of our pancreas.

Given what we know about certain enzymes and the pancreas, it should be easy to understand why someone with pancreatic cancer has a considerably more difficult (though certainly not impossible) challenge than those with other cancers. After all, the pancreas is what produces the enzymes, and if the pancreas itself is further impaired due to a malignant tumor growing on it, then its ability to produce important enzymes to suppress cancerous trophoblast cells is greatly compromised. But if someone has a malignant tumor elsewhere in the body – such as in the breast, prostate, or colon – assuming the pancreas still has some enzyme producing capability, the patient should have a relatively easier road to recovery.

ABSENCE OF ENOUGH PANCREATIC ENZYMES IS A DEFINITE RISK

A crucial question arises: why do we not have enough of these highly beneficial pancreatic enzymes in our bodies to digest the animal protein we eat and to keep ectopic germ cells that have been activated from becoming cancerous trophoblast cells? To a great extent, it is because we favor cooked foods (which are devoid of enzymes), and we tend not to eat many raw fruits and vegetables which would introduce more enzymes into our bodies.

If we significantly reduce our dietary intake of all animal products and significantly increase our intake of raw fruits and vegetables, we would surely supply our bodies with more vital enzymes and it would lessen the heavy demand placed on the pancreas to produce certain enzymes. We typically eat about twice as much animal protein as is necessary, and unfortunately, much of it is never fully digested and used by the body. Even most vegetables and many of the fruits that people eat are cooked. The pancreas then, has to try to produce the necessary enzymes; but over a period of time, that becomes quite a challenge. It is no wonder that we find that the pancreas in many people has become enlarged because, as we know, when a muscle in the body gets repeated workout it becomes enlarged. An overworked and often enlarged pancreas that starts to malfunction cannot secrete enough pancreatic enzymes to digest our food properly, nor can it supply enough of the same pancreatic enzymes to suppress potentially cancerous trophoblast cells. In short, our present diet places a great demand on the pancreas, and the challenge to this very important organ grows even more crucial as our bodies age and we continue nourishing it with foods lacking in enzymes.

Cooked animal protein presents a special problem for someone facing the challenges of cancer because it contains no enzymes of its own. The cooking of it kills the enzymes, and that requires the pancreas to have to work hard to produce the enzymes to digest it.

Those who discover that they have cancer who stop eating animal products and start consuming mainly raw foods can expect definite improvement at the cellular level, even if the cancer is discovered in an advanced stage.

If you remember only one thing from this book, it should be that the root cause of cancer, any cancer, relates to the body's inability to properly digest animal protein which stems from a failure of the pancreas to produce enough of certain digestive enzymes.

In addition to meat, most dairy products are also devoid of enzymes, because when dairy products are pasteurized (cooked) enzymes are killed. Other non-animal protein sources such as avocados, nuts, sprouts, blue green algae, coconut, whole grain and seeds are more easily digested. Unlike animal protein, these non-animal protein sources do not require the pancreas to produce large quantities of trypsin and chymotrypsin which are the main digestive enzymes necessary for digesting animal protein.

CANCER, A NATURAL PROCESS THAT MISFIRED, SENDING THE WRONG SIGNALS

When Dr. Beard, who was a professor of comparative embryology and Edinburgh University Medical School, began research into the cause of cancer in 1888, he focused mainly on the abnormal development of the human embryo (fertilized egg). In doing so, he determined that "cancer is a natural phenomenon, not a disease; although it may bring disease in its train."[4] He also noted with regret that the treatment of cancer was assigned not to scientific observers (such as embryologists) who discovered the origins and nature of the illness, but to physicians, most of whom believed it to be an incurable disease.

The idea that cancer could be a natural phenomenon probably seems incredible to most readers. We usually think of a natural phenomenon as something beneficial to us – such as the change of seasons or of the sun rising and setting. But we need to remember that some natural phenomena have non-beneficial effects on human life. Take for example earthquakes, volcanoes or hurricanes, all have the capability to destroy homes and kill thousands.

CANCER IS A PROCESS

It is a malfunction in the metabolic process, *pancreatic enzyme production* and distribution are out of order.

Cancer is NOT a malignant tumor, it is the malfuntioning PROCESS that produced the tumor.

Similarly, the natural phenomenon called cancer brings great pain; and although the cancer itself is not a disease, as Dr. Beard notes, it brings disease in its aftermath. An analogy might be heavy rains flooding a city causing sewers to back up, and thereby increasing the risk of the outbreak of disease. Fortunately, we have learned to take measures to prevent the risk of illness caused by flooding. Continuing our analogy, in the case of cancer there are also things we can do to avert the disease that otherwise follows.

In effect, cancer, no matter where it manifests in the body is part of a natural process, even though that process has misfired and set off false signals in the body to do the wrong thing at the wrong time and place. Dr. Beard and other researchers who have followed his line of inquiry determined that we can treat cancer by introducing the necessary pancreatic enzymes into our bodies, often with the help of medical professionals. However, we can also introduce the necessary pancreatic enzymes into our bodies through the food we eat.

MALIGNIN STIMULATES TUMOR CELL GROWTH

Fortunately, our bodies routinely destroy potentially cancerous cells daily, thanks to the action of circulating pancreatic enzymes. But if a malignant tumor does develop, it grows by feeding on surrounding tissue in the same way that trophoblast cells feed on the uteral tissue of a pregnant woman. In order to digest human protein tissue, the tumor mass makes its own enzyme called malignin. Malignin breaks down the surrounding good tissue and this enables the malignant tumor to grow; we can think of malignin as a tumor growth stimulator. Luckily, scientists have learned how to suppress the affects of malignin, thus preventing malignant tumor growth.

TRYPSIN ENZYMES HELP HALT TUMOR GROWTH

Dr. Beard learned that the enzyme trypsin is the mirror image of malignin (as the right and left hands are mirror images of each other), and that trypsin circulating in the body in sufficient quantities can nullify the malignin and thus suppress the growth of the malignant tumor. This discovery highlights once again the importance of insuring that pancreatic enzymes are always present in our bodies. Readers will be glad to know that enzymes that are very similar to trypsin and chymotrypsin enzymes are found in fresh pineapple and in papaya. Also, in some instances people have obtained patented drugs that contain trypsin and chymotrypsin. One such patented drug is called WOBE-MUGOS, and it has reportedly produced good results in preventing tumor growth.[5]

When trophoblast cells develop and start invading the surrounding good tissue, the cancerous process will continue; it will present increasingly serious health challenges unless it is halted with the introduction of pancreatic enzymes. Many people often refer to it as a "fight against cancer," because once this cancerous process is discovered, we must take immediate and aggressive action to change the chemistry in our bodies. Time is especially of the essence if the malignant tumor is in the pancreas, liver or stomach because all three organs contribute vitally to enzyme production and digestion.[7]

Cancer, then, is actually not the spreading lump that a woman discovers in her breast, or the malignant growth that the doctor discovers in a man's prostate. The malignant growth that we incorrectly call cancer (no matter where it is found) is in reality the symptom, not the disease itself. Malignant tumor removal is not equivalent to curing cancer. Again, all that is needed to create cancer (any cancer) in our bodies is a deficiency of pancreatic enzymes, particularly those that aid the digestion of animal protein.

Dr. Beard's discovery of the root cause of the disease that has come to be called the trophoblast theory of cancer, has received relatively little attention since he published his revolutionary work *The Enzyme Treatment of Cancer and Its Scientific Basis*, in London in 1911. And presently, it is not that health practitioners disagree with the trophoblastic explanation for the cause of cancer – in large part, they do not know about it because modern medicine focuses primarily on that which derives from cancer, the malignant tumor, and not on the underlying cause of the cancer itself.[7]

The Onset of Cancer and
Pregnancy Are Similar

We have demonstrated that cancer in males and females derives from trophoblast activity that went wrong. Since pregnancy also involves trophoblast activity, it is therefore crucial that we understand the nature of cancer well enough to distinguish between it and the onset of pregnancy. On November 19, 1999 the *Seattle Post-Intelligencer* newspaper printed an article about a 24-year-old woman who had been trying to get pregnant. After experiencing some bleeding, she went for a medical check-up and was tested for the presence of the human chorionic gonadotropic hormone, or hCG.

The presence of hCG is considered a strong indicator of pregnancy, but in the absence of certain other signs of pregnancy high hCG levels can also indicate cancer. It turns out that all trophoblast cells (whether they are in a pregnant woman or in someone with cancer) are covered with an outer coating of hCG, which can often be detected in the urine. If a person is either pregnant or has cancer, an hCG pregnancy test will help confirm either or both. The test is reported to be roughly 85 percent accurate. In the case of the young woman in the article, the results suggested cancer of the reproductive organs.

Based on their assessment, this woman's medical professionals thought the medical tests indicated cancer, so they treated her with chemotherapy for "trophoblast disease" when in fact, she had no such illness. The Post-Intelligencer article indicated that the outcome of this mistake had a profoundly negative impact on the young woman's health. Unfortunately, she has not been able to become pregnant and give birth. It is crucial that we understand the root cause of cancer to avoid confusing it with the onset of pregnancy and visa versa.

CANCER AND DIET

We can now state that what we commonly call "cancer" is actually millions of trophoblast cells following a misguided life cycle because they escaped being destroyed due to an absence of various pancreatic enzymes. We can help insure that our bodies have enough pancreatic enzymes by including in our daily diet raw foods that include onions, garlic, mustard, chilies, lima beans, black-eyed peas, apples, pears, and dark green leafy vegetables. High on the list are sprouted seeds (especially broccoli sprouts) and fresh fruits, including pineapples and papayas. In addition to other beneficial effects, these foods are loaded with live enzymes that our bodies sorely need, especially as we age and as our pancreas is increasingly challenged. In Chapter Eight, we will see that many of these foods contain an important naturally occurring ingredient called nitriloside (or amygdalin). A simple change of diet can greatly relieve some of the demand to produce enzymes otherwise placed on an overworked pancreas.

When we are under extensive stress, our body will produce metabolic enzymes to help us deal with it. When we challenge our body with things like breathing polluted air, drinking chlorinated water, overeating, using tobacco and not getting proper rest, our body has to produce enzymes to cope with their negative impact. Researchers have found that when the pancreas is greatly challenged, it often steals enzyme potential from other parts of the body, which causes other problems. Basically, we are at greatest risk of cancer when the pancreas is malfunctioning because of overwork.

Paulo Toniodo of the New York University Center conducted a case-control study to investigate the role of diet in breast cancer. The study compared the diets of 250 women with breast cancer with the diets of a random sample of 499 women from the general population. According to the completed questionnaires, women from the two groups ate about the same amount of all foods except animal products. What made the cancer patients different was that they had eaten more meat, cheese, butter and milk. Using a statistical technique called multivariate analysis, it was determined that women who consumed more animal products had up to three times the cancer risk of other women. The study showed that a dietary reduction in fat and proteins of animal origin can contribute to the substantial reduction in the incidence of breast cancer among groups who consume a lot of animal products.[8]

It is especially important that those facing the challenge of cancer obtain their protein from easily digestible sources, choosing protein-rich foods such as avocados, broccoli sprouts, coconut, blue green algae, and nuts, such as almonds, pecans, walnuts, and pistachios. Some health practitioners familiar with the enzyme therapy for cancer advocate that cancer patients consume no protein of any kind after 1:00 p.m. daily; the body's ability to properly digest and metabolize protein is greatest before midday.

As has been mentioned, the enzymes from fresh, uncooked fruits and vegetables are alive. They have not been killed like the enzymes in foods subjected to the heat of cooking. Daily consumption of living foods, especially wild berries, tomatoes, garlic, broccoli sprouts, mangos, papayas and pineapples and citrus, to mention just a few, can interrupt the cancer process.

The importance of consuming foods daily that contain their own enzymes cannot be over emphasized.

---

[3]John Beard, Doctor of Science. *The Enzyme Treatment of Cancer And Its Scientific Basis.* Copyright 1911. London Chatto & Windus. Also, see *The Unitarian or Trophoblastic Thesis of Cancer* by Ernst T. Krebs, Jr., Ernst T. Krebs Sr. and Howard H. Beard as printed in the Medical Record, 163:149-174, July 1950.

[4]John Beard, Doctor of Science. *The Enzyme Treatment of Cancer And Its Scientific Basis.* Copyright 1911. London Chatto & Windus. Page 39.

[5]For more information about this drug, contact your health care practitioner, and see Franz Klaschka's book *Oral Enzymes – New Approach to Cancer Treatment*, 1966, ISBN 3-910075-22-3.

[6]For more information, see *"The Unitarian or Trophoblastic Thesis of Cancer,"* by Ernst T. Krebs, Jr.; Ernst T. Krebs, Sr.; and Howard H. Beard in the July 1950 issue of the *Medical Record* (Volume 163, pp.149-74). See also *"Cancer or Cancers"* by Ernst T. Krebs, Jr., in the November 1946 issue of *California Medicine* (Volume 65, pp. 261-62). For additional information about the trophoblast theory of cancer, see the Robert Cathey Research Source at www.navi-net/~rsc.

[7]For another explanation of Dr. Beard's theory, see Dr. Robert Kelley's *One Answer to Cancer* (1998) and Professor Kathy P. Fairbanks' article, *"The Scientific Basis of the Kelley Metabolic Program."*

[8]To read the details of Paulo Toniolo's study, see *The Journal of the National Cancer Institute*, 1989 (Volume 81, pages 278-86).

CHAPTER 2 ⸻⸻⸻⸻⸻⸻⸻⸻⸻⸻

Cancer and Oxygen

"We can look at oxygen deficiency as the single greatest cause of disease."

– DR. STEPHEN LEVINE

SUMMARY:

It is very important to know the role of oxygen in the life of healthy cells, as well as it's role in cancerous cells. In addition, this chapter offers practical information about the basic nature of cancer cells. Finally, we look at the seldom discussed but crucial role of water in our bodies.

Dr. Otto Warburg received the Nobel Prize in 1931 for his discovery that, unlike other cells of the human body, cancer cells do not use oxygen. Cancer cells are anaerobic, which means they derive their energy without needing oxygen. Normal healthy cells burn oxygen and glucose (blood sugar) for energy, and they release carbon dioxide and water. These healthy cells function aerobically, which means they utilize oxygen in their production of energy.

Cancer cells, on the other hand, lack oxygen; yet they still produce energy (though inefficiently) by burning only glucose, and lots of it. This inefficient sugar burning process (called sugar fermentation) releases mainly lactic acid and carbon monoxide (instead of carbon dioxide). Cancer cells have to work harder and reproduce faster than healthy cells to produce energy from glucose, thriving in an environment of high sugar and high

---

CANCER CELLS

They produce energy from glucose alone, and require no oxygen. They thrive in an environment high in refined and processed sugar and high acidity. Because they use no oxygen, cancer cells reproduce very inefficiently and with great rapidity.

NORMAL HEALTHY CELLS

They burn oxygen and glucose to produce energy. Relative to cancer cells, this energy producing process is considerably more efficient. Most healthy cells do not do well in a highly acidic environment; they generally require a slightly alkaline pH, and a plentiful supply of oxygen to do their work.

acidity (remember that they produce lactic acid). So, as Nobel Prize-winning Dr. Warburg discovered in 1931, cancer cells can NOT exist in an environment that is high in oxygen, low in sugar, and where there is an alkaline pH (as opposed to a low acidic pH).

According to Dr. Warburg's findings, anyone who has a malignant tumor, or who wishes to prevent one, should find ways to oxygenate the tissues of the body. That is why aerobic exercises such as walking, stationary bicycling, swimming, or using treadmills and trampolines are all highly recommended, as is the deep breathing of fresh air. Some people have even done various aerobic exercises while breathing pure oxygen. Others make a conscious effort to do deep breathing as a way of getting more oxygen to the tissues. Some people choose to walk twice a day for at least twenty minutes each. Aerobic exercises move the lymph system around in the body, and this is important because many tissues depend on the lymph system to provide nutrients (including oxygen) and to carry off waste.

Chlorophyll and oxygen have a unique relationship. Chlorophyll contains magnesium, which carries oxygen to all parts of the body, and deep green leafy vegetables are by far the richest source of chlorophyll. Most other foods have little to no chlorophyll. This is one of many reasons why it is to the absolute benefit of anyone facing the challenge of cancer to drink four ounces of fresh squeezed juice from deep green leafy vegetables four times a day, and to eat these vegetables (uncooked) with their meals. (Incidentally, if green juice is too bitter when you first start on it, mix in a bit of fresh squeezed carrot and celery juice, and the juice from not more than a fourth of an apple).

Remember that it is especially important to ingest raw fruits and vegetables, as they are live foods whose enzymes have not been destroyed by cooking. In addition to being a superior source of nutrients, raw fruits and vegetables have a much higher water content than those that are cooked; and of course, water contains oxygen. So creating an oxygen-rich (aerobic) environment throughout the body strengthens the healthy cells while suppressing the growth of unhealthy (cancerous) cells. As a result, the immune system has a better chance to do its work of fighting the cancer. Another good reason to eat raw fruits and vegetables is that cancer cells are known to thrive in an acidic (or low pH) environment, and there is no better way to increase the pH or make the body more alkaline (and thus less inviting for cancerous growth) than by consuming deep green leafy vegetables. Read more about the importance of a proper alkaline balance in the next chapter.

As important as oxygen is to our bodies, it is also true that as we use it, sometimes its molecules become unstable. This happens when oxygen molecules lose an electron in their outer orbit and they go searching for one. These unstable oxygen molecules are called free radicals. They circulate in the body causing damage because they collide randomly with good molecules while searching for an electron to replace the missing one in their outer orbit. This damaging and haphazard action of free radicals is quite destabilizing. It can cause our bodies to age faster, and puts us at risk for contracting diseases.

The good news is antioxidant enzymes halt and reverse the debilitating action of free radicals. They provide an extra electron to give to free radicals, thus neutralizing their effects. Antioxidants include Vitamin C, Vitamin E, beta carotene, and selenium. Fresh uncooked fruits and vegetables (those that come in various colors of deep green, yellow, red, purple and orange) are excellent sources of antioxidants and antioxidant enzymes.

THE IMPORTANCE OF WATER

All functions of the body are regulated by the flow of water. Further, all monitoring systems (for example, the immune function) are based on the regulation of water, not on the regulation of solid matter or of hormones. It is water that regulates all functions of the body, and that delivers nutrients and removes toxic wastes; water also brings oxygen to all parts of the body. The hydrogen in water is essential for the movement of electrons throughout our body, and in turn for the creation of energy. These simple yet profound observations were made after in-depth study by London University trained physician, Dr. F. Batmanghelidj (pronounced "Batman-ge-lij") who has researched and written extensively about water in connection with various health challenges.

Both the nervous system and enzymes depend on water, the body's means of transport. As important as enzymes are, they could not get to where they need to be if there was no water to transport them. In effect, it is water that energizes all the chemical processes in the body. Our body is 75 percent water and our brain is 85 percent water. Dr. Batmanghelidj recommends that we drink at least eight glasses of water daily – not sodas, fruit juices, coffee, or milk – but water. He points out that without water, the lungs begin to shut down, and that is how asthma develops as a sign of progressive dehydration. Dr. Batmanghelidj's research confirms that adult onset diabetes is generally the result of prolonged lack of water consumption. It has been said that water is the most effective natural medicine for all life forms, and that it is the most effective "solvent" for both the inside and outside of the body. Medical practitioners are increasingly recognizing that chronic dehydration is often the beginning of what puts us at risk for degenerative diseases.

Dr. Batmanghelidj observed that somewhere around the age of twenty-five we start losing our sense of thirst; in other words, our critical perception that our body needs water decreases as we age. And by not recognizing this need, we tend to become more and more dehydrated as years go by. An added benefit of water is that the hydrogen within it helps move the body chemistry toward a more alkaline pH, a subject discussed in greater detail in the next chapter.

Finally, as vital as oxygen is for preventing and recovering from cancer, if water was not available, oxygen could not do its work. If some area of the body does not receive much water, that area cannot benefit from oxygen. In that respect, water is even more important than oxygen. And think about this for a moment: mainstream medicine depends heavily on the intravenous drip, which is simply water (and some sort of sugar or saline solution) introduced directly into the veins.[9] One can go to any hospital on any given day and discover that a large number of patients are hooked up to intravenous water intake. Why then should we wait until people are sick to give them the simple remedy of water? Instead, Dr. Batmanghelidj would urge that we each give ourselves adequate water each day – at least eight glasses along with a pinch of sea salt to maintain health. (I can state unequivocally that adequate water has recently been the cure for a lower back problem that I previously endured off and on since the mid 1960s).

---

[9] F. Batmanghelidj, M.D. *Water: The Immune Breakthrough & Pain and Cancer "Wonder Drug"*. This was from a March 19, 1992 lecture given by the author, who conducted research for twenty years on the function of water in the body.

Alkalize For Your Health

Man is not nourished by what he swallows,
but by what he digests and uses.

– HIPPOCRATES

SUMMARY:

We often eat foods that contribute to making our
body chemistry more acidic, and an acidic environment
can be conducive to cancerous growth. Learn more
about that as you read the next few pages.

Many years ago chemists devised a scale of 0 to 14 to measure something they called the relative acidity and alkalinity of a solution. By that scale, it was decided that a solution would be considered acid if it measured between zero up to but not including seven. If the solution measured seven, it would be considered neutral. And if it measured more than seven and up to fourteen, the solution would be said to be alkaline. The scale measures the percentage of hydrogen in the solution, so it was designated the "pH" scale, which stands for "percent hydrogen". See the pH Scale on page 38.

It has long been established that certain parts of our body are designed to function best in an alkaline environment. One such area is the blood. Blood seeks to maintain itself at 7.4, or slightly alkaline, on the pH scale. Through a process of homeostasis, the body endeavors to maintain the blood at that pH level. This means that our bodies will do whatever is necessary to keep the blood as close to 7.4 as possible. To accomplish this, it sometimes has to rob alkaline potential from other parts of the body; while this helps maintain the desired alkalinity of the blood, it (unfortunately) changes the pH of the part of the body that was robbed, thus making it less alkaline and more acidic.

One part of the body from which the blood will steal alkaline potential is the mouth, or oral cavity. When that happens, the mouth becomes more acidic, often resulting in cavities and diseased gums. Another unfortunate result of our body's having to steal alkaline potential from the mouth is that it changes our taste buds causing them to have a strong preference for acid forming foods, and a dislike for foods that are alkaline.

That is why fresh deep green leafy vegetables such as collard greens, mustard greens, spinach, kale, chard, or bok choy are less often included in shoppers' carts at the grocery checkout stand. And when they are purchased they are generally not consumed with the same regularity and eagerness as other cooked and processed foods. As a result, our body chemistry is often acidic because we eat too many acid forming foods and not enough alkaline forming foods.

It has long been known that our bodies function best when we consume approximately 25 percent acid forming foods and approximately 75 percent alkaline forming foods. But in fact, most of us in the Western World have those recommended figures inverted; that is, we consume approximately 75 percent acid forming foods and about 25 percent alkaline forming foods.

It has been established clinically that malignant tumors or cancer cells require an acidic environment. They cannot gain a foothold and thrive in an alkaline environment. It is important to understand that the acidic pH of cancer cells decreases the oxygen carrying ability of the surrounding blood. We saw in the previous chapter that cancer cells thrive in an environment where there is a lack of oxygen. How then can we make a highly acidic body more alkaline? Deep breathing exercises can help, and eating foods that are alkaline forming is another way. In that respect, there is no better food than uncooked deep green leafy vegetables.

Alkaline forming foods include nearly all raw fruits and vegetables. Acid forming foods include nearly all cooked fruits and vegetables, pasteurized foods, grains, all cooked meats, nuts, and most dairy products. In addition, emotions such as excessive worry and stress have an acidic effect on the body. Consider our modern lifestyle where we are often under stress and where our typical diet is heavily weighted in favor of cooked and refined foods, animal products, and grains. Is it any wonder that our overall body chemistry is often more acidic than it should be? As a result, our blood is critically challenged to try to maintain an alkaline pH of 7.4. And given this situation, our overall body chemistry as measured by our saliva and urine is often too acidic to support good health. According to Dr. Patrick Quillin in *Beating Cancer With Nutrition*, the acceptable pH for saliva is 6.0 to 7.5, and for urine is 4.5 to 8.4.

An unfavorably acidic environment is where primitive ectopic germ cells that we referred to in Chapter one can become trophoblast, or cancerous cells, and if there is also an absence of circulating pancreatic enzymes the tumor grows virtually unchecked.

It is very important to observe a lifestyle and dietary regimen that ensures an alkaline environment in the body along with an abundance of circulating pancreatic enzymes.

It is actually possible to measure your own pH level (alkalinity/acidity level) with the use of specially treated paper purchased at a pharmacy. This paper can also be obtained through mail order; one source is Micro Essential Laboratory, Inc., in Brooklyn, New York. The best time to do this test, which involves testing your saliva and urine, is just after you arise in the morning.

Based on my research, it is clear that normalizing the alkaline/acid chemistry is absolutely key to creating an environment that is uninviting to cancer. Since we are on the subject of acidity in the body, it should also be noted that almost all patented medicines and prescription drugs and over the counter drugs have the effect of making the body chemistry more acidic.

In a place such as southern India, where almost everyone eats a simple diet of rice, lentils and yogurt, there is very little cancer. Clearly, they eat a far greater proportion of alkaline-forming foods. True, the people there may suffer from poverty, as well as from related problems of malnutrition, high infant mortality, and contagious diseases, but degenerative conditions such as cancer, diabetes and heart problems are almost entirely absent.

It is vitally important that we alkalize in order to support good health at the cellular level, therefore making our bodies uninviting places for the incubation of malignant tumors.

PH SCALE

acidic   *alkaline*

0 ———————————— 7 ———————————— 14

On the pH scale, "0" is extremely acidic, and 14 is extremely alkaline. 6.9 would be considerd very mildly acidic, and 7.4 is considered mildly alkaline. 7 is neutral. Water has a pH of 7.

A Strong Immune System is Key

"The best prescription is knowledge."

— Dr. C. Everett Koop,
former Surgeon General
of the United States

Summary:

We will learn in this chapter what the immune system is, why it is important in connection with the challenge of cancer. We will discuss things we can do to boost the immune system, and will explain why sometimes the immune system is unable to successfully defend against cancer.

The importance of a strong immune system cannot be overemphasized. Some have called it the first line of defense against everything from the common cold to AIDS and cancer. It is the immune system that destroys cancer cells – that is, when it can locate them. As we will see, unfortunately, cancer cells develop strategies, or escape mechanisms, to flee from the effects of the immune system. That is all the more reason why the immune system always needs to be in tip top shape.

In simple terms, the immune system is a group of cells, biochemicals, tissues and organs strategically located throughout the body to help protect it against foreign invaders. A healthy lifestyle is the best way to maintain a strong and vibrant immune system. A balanced diet, exercise, adequate sleep and maintaining a positive outlook all provide the best defense. In that regard, there are two simple facts that virtually everyone knows, but too few heed: you cannot be healthy without a balanced diet, and you cannot have a balanced diet without deep green leafy vegetables.

These facts are so obvious, yet all too often people refuse to act as if they matter. One common denominator that exists in the vast majority of diseased people is mineral deficiency, and this deficiency can be easily corrected by simply getting back to basics and consuming living and green foods.

A living food is one that is uncooked, non-pasteurized, minimally processed and therefore contains an enzyme complex capable of digesting itself and contributing excess enzymes to relieve stress at the cellular level. We saw in Chapter One of this book that Dr. Beard did pioneering work on the cause of cancer, discovering that it was a deficiency in our body's ability to produce certain pancreatic enzymes. Raw deep green leafy vegetable are capable of supplying many of those enzymes, and no further clinical studies are needed as proof.

Dr. Virginia C. Livingston, a recognized pioneer in successfully employing natural means of addressing cancer, practiced internal medicine until her death in 1990. She points out that: "One of the most vital systems of the body that cannot be sustained by devitalized, dead food is the immune system."

Research has confirmed that there are steps we can take to boost our immune system's capabilities:

■ Get enough rest. Try for seven to eight hours of sleep a day. This is especially important if one is under stress.

■ Exercise regularly. The beneficial effects of exercise are numerous and well known. For the cancer patient, exercise has been shown to help distribute oxygen to all tissues of the body. Malignant tumor cells, as we have seen, do not thrive on oxygen; in fact, it has been shown in the lab that oxygen contributes to their shutting down.

■ Drink plenty of good pure water (not coffee, juice, soft drinks, or caffeine tea), no less than eight glasses daily. Among other things, water helps flush toxins out of the body. Also, and very importantly, adequate water prevents the body from producing excessive histamine, which otherwise suppresses the immune system.

■ Consume fresh, uncooked fruits and vegetables daily. In addition to fresh fruits and vegetables, eat minimally processed foods such as broccoli sprouts, mung bean sprouts, whole grain such as oatmeal, millet, rye, flaxseed meal. Sprouts, as well as avocados, coconuts and nuts (almonds, pistachios, walnuts, pecans, but not peanuts), are good sources of protein.

■ Eat foods such as brown rice, lentils, and baked

yams. Also include in your diet foods such as garlic, turmeric, curry, ginger root and cabbage, and maitake and shitake mushrooms. These have all been shown to boost the immune system.

■ Maintain a joyful attitude, and practice prayer and/or meditation to cultivate and maintain an awareness of a Higher Power.

WHY CAN'T THE IMMUNE SYSTEM KILL CANCER CELLS?

For a good many years, scientists wondered why the immune system does not always destroy cancerous (or unhealthy) cells, since its main function is to get rid of harmful influences in the body. One of the things that Dr. Beard's research and others that followed him revealed was that cancerous (or trophoblast) cell tissue contains a protein and starchy coating that effectively disguises it to the immune system, making it "look" like good tissue that should be allowed to continue growing. This protein/starchy coating is part of the cancer cell's escape mechanism. But the enzyme amylase and other pancreatic enzymes such as trypsin and chymotrypsin can dissolve this protein/starchy coating, thus exposing the cancerous tissue so that the immune system is then able to recognize the cancerous tissue as an unhealthy influence that must be destroyed. If the body's immune function has not been suppressed, it will then destroy the cancerous tissue.

Let us restate in different words the vitally important point made in the above paragraph. Suppose you are in a city looking for a certain street. To find that street, you look for a street sign. When the immune function looks for a malignant tumor in the body it too looks for a sign , or "marker" on the surface of the malignant tumor. The markers are called antigens. These antigens let the immune system know that the tissue is malignant tumor and needs to be destroyed. But, unfortunately, malignant tumors can become encapsulated in a protein and starchy covering, and this protective coating effectively "hides" the cancer cell from the immune system. At other times tumor cells can be covered in red blood cells, which can also hide them from the immune system.

Fortunately, researchers discovered that the right enzyme complex can dissolve the protective coating from around the cancerous tissue and enable the immune system to "see" the unhealthy cancerous tissue and destroy it. We saw in Chapter One that it is important that our bodies have adequate circulating pancreatic enzymes (including amylase, trypsin, chymotrypsin and lipase) to combine with cancer cells to suppress their growth. Very importantly, that means consuming fresh squeezed deep green leafy vegetable juices, and pineapple and papaya juices; do this three or four times a day if the cancer is far advanced because they are known to contain the all important pancreatic enzymes for dissolving the protective coatings from around the cancer cells. Finally, assuming the immune system has not been suppressed, it will target and destroy the cancerous cells once they are exposed as unhealthy tissue. That is why a strong immune system is key.

The Healing Power of Deep Green Foods

"A man may esteem himself happy when that
which is his food is also his medicine."

– Henry David Thoreau

As we saw in Chapter One, cancer involves the changing of a primitive ectopic cell into an ectopic trophoblast cell. Cancer is actually a process that evidences a malignant tumor that grows and often spreads throughout the body. The malignant tumor (regardless of where it manifests) is merely the symptom of the cancerous process, it (the tumor mass) is the outcome of newly transformed trophoblast cells that are somehow doing the wrong thing at the wrong time and in the wrong place. It is important to remember from Chapter One that ectopic trophoblast cells do not develop spontaneously. They are part of the life cycle of primitive ectopic germ cells circulating in our bodies, and for various reasons these cells became activated and thus cancerous.

Cancer incubates for months and sometimes years before it manifests as a full-blown malignant tumor that can be detected by a medical scan procedure. We must make it our business to create an environment in the body where cancer cannot incubate and gain a foothold. If the cancerous process has already gained a foothold, we must then be especially aggressive and do things to break the cycle that allows the ectopic trophoblast cells to multiply.[10]

Interrupting cancer's incubation cycle is a tall order; but make no mistake – our bodies in practically every instance are up to the task. But it requires dietary and lifestyle changes. We have to eat a well rounded diet everyday that involves portions of uncooked deep green leafy vegetables – not vitamin pills or super food additives, but uncooked deep green leafy vegetables such as collard greens, mustard greens, turnip greens, kale, spinach and the green leaves of bok choy. For the cancer patient and for those who wish to prevent cancer, there are probably no more beneficial foods. The healing power of deep green leafy vegetables is unmatched by nutritional supplements or by medicines that mainly suppress symptoms. And speaking of symptoms, if the oil indicator light in your car came on (indicating your car is low in oil) the smart thing would be to add oil, and NOT to suppress the symptom by unscrewing the oil indicator bulb and pretending that all is well!

Without a doubt, it is best that the green foods be organically grown in soils rich in minerals. Unfortunately, it is often difficult to obtain such foods, and once they are found they are always more spendy. Here then is a strong argument for growing some of your own food, even if itís only sprouts grown in your kitchen window, or garlic and tomatoes grown in the flower bed. If someone cannot obtain organically grown foods all the time, they are still far better off eating commercially grown fruits and vegetables (or better yet, those from a farmer's market) as opposed to cooked, processed and denatured foods that come with no enzymes to facilitate digestion, and are greatly lacking in nutrient content.

THERE ARE ESSENTIALLY FIVE REASONS
WHY DEEP GREEN LEAFY VEGETABLES ARE SO
CRUCIAL TO GOOD HEALTH:

■ They are abundant in chlorophyll, which oxygenates the body. This feature alone is important to someone with cancer concerns, because, as we have seen, malignant tumors cannot thrive in an oxygen-rich environment. Uncooked green vegetables have an abundance of enzymes that rejuvenate the body and are responsible for carrying out virtually every chemical reaction at the cellular level. We saw in Chapter One that certain enzymes are necessary for dissolving the coating from around cancerous cells so the immune system can "see" them to destroy them. It is true that our bodies can produce enzymes, but they have a limited capability to do so. That is why it is important that we help our bodies by consuming foods that have their own live enzymes capable of aiding in the digestion of that food, and that even have excess enzymes that can combat the growth of activated ectopic trophoblast cells. The uncooked deep green leafy vegetable is such a food (I eat two or more servings of it daily, and drink a six-ounce glass of fresh green juice about three times a week).

THE MIRACLE OF CHLOROPHYLL

Chlorophyll is one of the more unique and powerfully beneficial substances in our diet. It contains magnesium, which makes possible the carrying of oxygen throughout the body. Chlorophyll is found only in green vegetables – the deeper the green the more chlorophyll. Oxygen is essential for good cellular health, an that's why chlorophyll is key.

■ These green vegetables have the ability to alkalize, to neutralize acids and to balance the pH. This ability to alkalize is undoubtedly one of the most powerful effects that interrupts the incubation of cancer-causing substances that begin with over acidity. As we have seen, it is crucial to good health that certain parts of our body be in an alkaline pH. One such example is the blood, which seeks to maintain a 7.4 (or slightly alkaline) pH. We have also seen that malignant tumors thrive in an acidic pH, and that they cannot survive in an alkaline pH. Accordingly, it is very important that we live a lifestyle and consume foods that alkalize certain parts of our body chemistry. Incidentally, doctors rarely raise the issue of the proper acid/alkaline balance in the body, probably because their focus is more directly on symptoms, and not so much on diet and the functioning of the body at the cellular level. That is all the more reason, however, why we each must make it our business to address this all-important area of the proper acid/alkaline balance.

■ Deep green leafy vegetables are an abundant source of trace minerals. A deficiency of trace minerals is said to be the main cause of most diseases today. In addition, they provide an abundance of calcium, a mineral that our bodies need in greater amounts, especially as we age. It is important to note that all of the vital nutrients in fresh green foods are bio-available, meaning that they are easily and readily assimilated into the body. You do not have to be concerned about taking a toxic dose of green foods (as you would with certain vitamin and mineral supplements), because any of their nutrients that the body does not need at the time are excreted through normal elimination. This is not the case with many supplements, excess amounts of which can be toxic.

■ Deep green leafy vegetables introduce light-weight vegetable protein into the body, which enhances the immune system and provides building blocks for lean connective tissue. This in turn strengthens the body, enabling it to withstand the physical stresses placed on it. Malignant tumors rob body tissue of vital protein, but as lightweight vegetable proteins are immediately available from deep green leafy vegetables, they can help maintain the muscle tissue, thus preventing the body from becoming greatly weakened.

In addition to the four main points just mentioned, deep green leafy vegetables are unique in that they actually make all the other foods we eat work better. That is, they act as catalysts to facilitate digestion (mainly through enzyme action), and facilitate the excretion of wastes by providing vital cell salts in the form of trace minerals. These foods also enable our bodies to have more energy, not because of their calories, because green foods do not have calories. Instead, they alkalize the small intestine, thus making it possible for the body to pass glucose through the intestinal barrier and to use the energy that had otherwise been stored as fat.

When it comes to whole foods such as green vegetables, nature weaves an intricate and interdependent mosaic. All of the nutrients in these foods are interdependent. Therefore you cannot get the full benefit from chlorophyll, enzymes, or trace minerals by isolating them into separate pills or capsules, because they depend on each other for proper assimilation into the body.

In summary, these green foods alkalize and oxygenate the body, strengthen the immune system, and provide vitally needed trace minerals, enzymes, plus lightweight protein. Obviously, they are not the only foods our bodies need, they are unique because they make all the other foods work better; plus they provide chlorophyll, and no other food has chlorophyll. Deep green leafy vegetables have been providing these benefits to the human body for countless centuries, long before there was any such thing as a clinical study. The good news is that these foods are all available from the produce section of most supermarkets, or even better, they can be made available from your own garden. It's particularly good if they can be organically grown, but if you can obtain only non-organically grown deep green leafy vegetables, by all means get them, because their healing power is profound.

It's important to remember, however, that changing your diet cannot undo or fully interrupt the cancer cycle overnight. Therefore, do not expect immediate, dramatic change when you start consuming a natural diet with a high percentage of raw unprocessed foods. Be prepared to stick with the new diet and lifestyle religiously for at least forty-five days or longer. The change will be gradual, almost unnoticeable at first, but it will occur.

---

[10]Some of the information in this chapter was adapted from the audio cassette tape, "The Healing Miracle of Green Foods" by David Sandoval of the G.K.C. Corporation in Long Beach, California.

Enzymes –
The Spark of Life

"All life processes take place through the action of ferments (enzymes), and without these there would be no life, such as we know it."

– John Beard, *The Enzyme Treatment of Cancer And Its Scientific Basis*, 1911

Consult almost any book on nutrition and you will learn the importance of getting adequate amounts of vitamins, minerals, and roughage in the diet. But often missing from the discussion is the topic of enzymes – those valuable nutrients that sustain life and rejuvenate cells by controlling virtually every chemical reaction that takes place in the body. Think of enzymes as the workers in our body, and proteins, vitamins, and minerals as the builders. To build a healthy structure we need both workers and builders. Trying to function without all the necessary enzymes is like trying to build a house all by yourself in one day.

Dr. Edward Howell, a widely recognized expert on enzymes, did more work in this area than practically any other scientist or physician in the twentieth century. In his seminal publication, *Enzyme Nutrition*, copyrighted 1985, Dr. Howell states the following:

"Enzymes are substances that make life possible. They are needed for every chemical reaction that takes place in the human body. No mineral, vitamin, or hormone can do any work without enzymes. Our bodies, all our organs, tissues, and cells, are run by metabolic enzymes. They are manual workers that build our body from protein, carbohydrates, and fats, just as construction workers build our homes. You may have all the raw materials with which to build, but without the workers (enzymes) you cannot even begin."

Anthony Cichoke, D.C., sums it up best when he says in his book *Enzymes and Enzyme Therapy* that: "Nothing (in the body) can take place without energy, and energy cannot be used or produced without enzymes."

ENZYMES, THE REAL WORKERS

Without them, vitamins and minerals are useless, and energy cannot be produced.

We are born with a finite and limited enzyme producing capability, so we must augment that by consuming enzyme-rich foods daily.

Low enzyme activity in the body brings on aging, degerative diseases (including cancer), and untimely death.

Many textbooks on the subject state that enzymes enter into chemical reactions in our body and influence those reactions, but are themselves not used up in the process.   Dr. Howell's extensive research, however, does not support that assertion. He makes it clear that we are born with a bank of enzymes, a certain enzyme potential (or "bank account"), and when that bank account is depleted the human body begins to age rapidly, and is more vulnerable to degenerative diseases, including cancer.

Research shows that enzymes actually perform the work of the body, and if they are not replaced they can become used up or worn out, and when that happens it puts our health on a rapid downhill path. It is therefore vital that we each make regular deposits to our enzyme bank account[11]. We can do that by eating primarily uncooked foods that have their own enzymes, as opposed to cooked foods, because the enzymes in cooked foods have been destroyed by the heat. Their enzymes are killed anytime foods are fried, baked, canned, dried, or irradiated. We should also understand that while some substances such as vitamins and minerals help make enzymes work better, there are other substances (including most medicines, and even aspirin) that suppress our body's enzymes[12].

TWO MAIN CATEGORIES OF ENZYMES

First, there are metabolic enzymes that are present in every cell, tissue, and organ, and that act as biochemical catalysts to control virtually every chemical reaction associated with our metabolism; and secondly, we have digestive enzymes, classified either as intrinsic (those that the body manufactures and secretes), or as extrinsic (those that come from raw fruits, vegetables, nuts and seeds). Fresh grown food contains enough active enzymes to digest the proteins, carbohydrates, or fats found in that food, and this makes digestion of these raw foods much easier when our body does not have to supply the digestive enzymes.

Fortunately, it is not necessary for someone to have a degree in biochemistry to understand the importance of enzymes. Aside from simply understanding that enzymes are vital to the body, the main thing we all need to remember is that when we cook a food above 122 degrees Fahrenheit, we permanently destroy its enzymes. Likewise, when we store foods at temperatures below 32 degrees Fahrenheit, their enzymes become inactive; but once the frozen food is thawed out the enzymes (if they were not killed before freezing the food) come alive again. To keep enzymes active, food should be kept at temperatures between 32 and 104 degrees Fahrenheit.

WE MUST EAT MORE LIVE FOODS THAT CONTAIN ENZYMES

Since the typical Western diet consists of about 90 percent cooked food, this means that we depend heavily on the intrinsic digestive enzymes (that is, the enzymes that our bodies produce) to help break down our food. As a result, we are continually depleting the body's enzyme bank account, while not making many deposits to that account. In addition, our bodies must also manufacture metabolic enzymes to help us through situations involving stress, anger, fear, and other strong emotions.

The pancreas is the principal organ that produces enzymes to aid the digestion of protein, fats, and carbohydrates. The enzymes that digest proteins are referred to as proteolytic enzymes, those that digest fats are called lipase enzymes, and those that digest carbohydrates (or starch) are called amylase enzymes. All three types are called pancreatic enzymes, since they are secreted by the pancreas.

As has been noted, since we typically consume very few foods that have their own enzymes, the pancreas therefore gets quite a workout day after day, year after year. We could ease this situation and undoubtedly extend the useful life of our pancreas simply by consuming more raw and uncooked foods and fewer processed and refined foods. In addition to eating fruits and vegetables, we also do a great service to our bodies when we consume protein-rich foods from plants that digest easily, such as fresh avocados, sprouts from broccoli or alfalfa or mung bean seeds, coconuts, blue green algae. Deep green leafy vegetables have an abundance of easily digested lightweight vegetable protein, along with valuable enzymes that are readily usable for helping build lean, strong muscular tissue.

Obviously, some of our food will be cooked, such as lentils, yams, lima beans, brown rice, black eye peas and some whole grains. Here is where one is well advised to consume them along with a high quality digestive enzyme supplement, preferably in powder form. Or better yet, eat them

---

". . . if uncooked food is eaten, fewer of your body's internal digestive enzymes will be called upon to perform the digestive function. That is, the body adapts to the plentiful supply of enzymes in the uncoooked foods by secreting less of its own digestive enzymes – this preserves your internal enzyme supplies for the important work of maintaining metabolic harmony."[13]

Enzyme Nutrition, p. 51,
copyright 1985,
by Dr. Edward Howell

---

with sprouts because live sprouts offer an abundance of enzymes. Again, the idea of the enzymes is to facilitate digestion by easing the demand that would otherwise be placed on the pancreas.

For someone facing the challenge of cancer, fresh enzyme-rich foods are particularly beneficial not only for their ease of digestion, but because, as we have mentioned, they supply excess enzymes that help suppress cancerous tumors. Papaya and pineapple are unique because they have been shown to provide proteolytic or protein digesting enzymes.

The enzyme from papaya is called papain and that from the pineapple is called bromelain. Bromelain is most concentrated in the skin and stem of the pineapple, so it is recommended that one not peel the pineapple, but instead process the juice from one-half of a pineapple each day through a slow speed 80 rpm juicer and drink the juice. The enzyme papain from papaya is also vital in helping suppress cancerous cells by working in concert with the enzyme amylase to dissolve the protective coating from around the cancerous cells. A half of a papaya should also be juiced daily for someone with cancer.

TRYPSIN AND CHYMOTRYPSON, CRUCIAL FOR PROTEIN DIGESTION

The enzymes trypsin and chymotrypsin are necessary for digesting animal protein (but not vegetable protein), and they have to be mainly manufactured by the pancreas, since we get none of these enzymes from the cooked meat. Papaya, pineapple, guava, kiwi and figs are known to contain animal protein digesting enzymes. Also, these enzymes (trypsin and chymotrypsin) have sometimes been gotten from pigs and taken in capsule form.

The subject of enzymes and their relation to our health is quite complex, but for the most part, if one observes a diet with a high percentage of raw fruits, vegetables, and nuts, then getting enough enzymes is not a problem. If for some reason you do not get enough enzymes through the foods you eat, there is a patented multi-enzyme complex tablet called Wobenzym that may be helpful. Wobenzym, according to information found at the website www.handpen.com, contains the following per tablet: 100 mg of pancreatin, 60 mg of papain, 45 mg of bromelain, 24 mg of trypsin, 1 mg of chymotrypsin, and 50 mg of rutosid.

Consult a health food store and your health practitioner for further information about this product. Remember, however, that digestive enzymes that break down protein can be obtained from consuming pineapple, papaya, figs, guava, and kiwi. But if you feel you do not get enough of them, then perhaps an enzyme supplement might be considered. A small firm that specializes in digestive enzyme supplements is The Mineral Connection (glyndak@yahoo.com) near Austin, Texas, they can be reached at 1-800-742-2560.

If a malignant tumor has already developed, it would be wise to consult with a health practitioner who is competent in the area of enzyme treatment of cancer. The Cancer Cure Foundation is a non-profit entity that can recommend health practitioners in this area.

Franz Klaschka, a highly respected German doctor, authored *Oral Enzymes – New Approach to Cancer Treatment* (Grafelfing, Germany: Forum-Med.-Verl. Ges.,1966, ISBN 3-910075-22-3).

In his book, he writes about the successful treatment of cancer using an enzyme product called Wobe Mugos, each tablet of which contains 100 mg of papain, 40 mg of trypsin, and 40 mg of chymotrypsin (according to the website at www.handpen.com). The enzyme treatment of cancer has produced good results in recent years, and is especially encouraging because it is not invasive (like surgery), does not introduce poisons into the body, and does not depress the immune system, as is the case with chemotherapy and radiation.

Dr. Klaschka's publication cites 383 research findings in the areas of cancer, enzymes, and the immune function. He notes in the introduction to his book that Scottish scientist Dr. John Beard reported remarkable successes in treating cancer patients with pancreatic enzymes from fresh piglet and lamb pancreases.

Unfortunately, Dr. Beard's studies fell into oblivion during most of the 1900s before a reliable protocol could be established to insure that the enzymes from piglets and lambs did not spoil or lose their effectiveness due to poor storage and handling procedures. But the problem of enzyme storage and handling has been solved, and the enzyme treatment of cancer, administered through trained health care practitioners, is significantly benefiting ever greater numbers of patients.

NUTS AS A SOURCE OF PROTEIN

It is commonly known that various nuts are a good source of protein, they are more easily digested than cooked animal protein. However, there is something about the enzyme composition of nuts that is different from that of fruits and vegetables, and we need to be aware of it. Nuts such as pecans, almonds, walnuts, filberts, pistachios, brazil nuts, etc. all contain "enzyme inhibitors" in order to restrict (or inhibit) enzyme activity until the particular nut (or seed) falls to the ground and is moistened by the earth so that it can germinate and sprout a new plant.

In other words, nature devised a way to keep the enzymes of nuts inactive (by inhibiting them) until such time as the nut (or seed) is ready to start growing into another pecan tree or walnut tree, etc. So when we eat nuts, since their enzymes have been restricted or inhibited, we have to be sure to chew them well in order to release the otherwise inhibited enzymes.

Dr. Edward Howell would say that anytime we eat substantial quantities of nuts, there is one of two things we should do in order to facilitate their proper digestion: either take an enzyme supplement at the time the nuts are eaten, or soak them in water for 24 to 36 hours and let nature begin the germination process of releasing (or uninhibiting) the enzymes to help with digestion. Similarly, Dr. Kelley in his book *One Answer To Cancer* makes the point that if seeds and nuts are either chewed well or soaked overnight, this reduces the effect of the enzyme inhibitors and makes the seed or nut more readily digestible.

Finally, enzymes are so essential to good health that we should not wait for health practitioners to recommend them for treating our illnesses. Instead, we should "treat" ourselves to them every day in the normal course of nourishing our bodies with enzyme-rich foods.

---

[11]Dr. Edward Howell. *Enzyme Therapy: The Food Enzyme Concept.* Copy right 1985. Avery, a member of Penguin Putnam Inc.

[12]*Enzymes: Are You Getting Enough?* by Anthony J. Cichoke. *Better Nutrition Magazine.* March 2000.

[13]Dr. Edward Howell. *Enzyme Therapy: The Food Enzyme Concept.* Copyright 1985. p. 51. Avery, a member of Penguin Putnam Inc.

CHAPTER 7 _____

Cancer and Foods

"Your food shall be your remedies, and your remedies shall be your food."

— HIPPOCRATES

In 1997 an international panel of 15 scientists from nine countries assessed hundreds of studies on diet and cancer. In their published report issued by the World Cancer Research Fund they offer fifteen specific points of advice to the reader; and the first is that we should "...choose predominantly plant-based diets rich in a variety of vegetables and fruits, legumes and minimally processed starchy staple foods."[14]

Most people know that deep green vegetables such as broccoli, spinach, collard greens, and kale are strong cancer fighters. What is less well known is that certain foods are conducive to cancer in that they create an environment where malignant tumors can thrive. If you have cancer, you will want to consider AVOIDING: sugar (fructose, sucrose, brown sugar as well), aspartame (found in NutriSweet or Equal), sucralose (also known as Spenda and is a sweetener), all trans fatty acids, MSG (this spice is often included in prepared foods and is not listed), and white flour and other foods made from refined grains. Simple carbohydrates, refined sugar, refined flour, and most of the oils commonly used in cooking all foster an environment in the body that is very friendly to the growth of cancerous tissue. In addition, fragmented (or refined) foods, as well as those containing preservatives, coloring, and various synthetic chemicals cannot possibly contribute to a healthy cellular environment in the body. It cannot be emphasized strongly enough that white sugar and white flour should be off limits for someone facing cancer because these are two foods on which fast-growing cancer cells thrive. Certainly, the fifteen professionals that prepared the above-mentioned Report on cancer and nutrition would concur with this.

Anyone facing cancer and who is serious about wanting to overcome it will want to consider giving up meat altogether, and focus more on a plant-based diet involving uncooked fruits and vegetables. The American Cancer Society in its nutrition guidelines stresses plant sources as the primary basis for nourishment. One of the problems with meat protein is that the same scarce protein digesting enzymes required for digesting the meat are needed for digesting (or dissolving) the protective protein and starchy coating from around the cancer cells. Another reason for avoiding meat is that it contains female sex hormones. Commercially produced beef, and poultry are injected by the farmers with large quantities of hormones of various kinds. As was noted in Chapter One, an imbalance of female sex hormones is one factor that activates ectopic germ cells causing them to convert to trophoblast (or cancerous) cells. Even soy products, unless fermented or sprouted, are not the best protein substitutes. Soy has enzyme inhibitors that block the action of trypsin and other enzymes needed for protein digestion. In addition, soybeans contain hemagglutinin, a clot promoting substance that causes red blood cells to clump together.

One is far better off satisfying their body's need for protein by eating avocados, uncooked deep green leafy vegetables, and sprouts from the sprouted seeds of broccoli, mung beans, radish.

Protein can also be obtained from nuts such as almonds, sunflower seeds, walnuts, cashews, pecans, brazil nuts, filberts, seeds, and pistachios, although nuts should be chewed thoroughly and/ or soaked as was mentioned above. Dr. William Kelley recommends anyone facing the challenge of cancer only eat protein foods for breakfast and lunch, because in that way the pancreatic enzymes used in the digestion of the protein are used for only about six hours out of each day. This leaves some eighteen hours each day for producing enzymes that dissolve the protein and starchy coating from around the cancer cells, in order to expose the cancer cells to the immune system.

Except for raw goat milk, regular pasteurized milk and dairy need to be avoided if you have cancer. Pasteurized milk has no enzymes to facilitate digestion, and this is a problem for a cancer patient whose body is already challenged in trying to produce enough protein digesting enzymes to suppress the tumor. Also, there are female sex hormones in dairy products that are believed to promote cancer.

It is widely known that hydrogenated and processed oils of all kind are not good for cancer patients, they further contribute to a friendly environment for cancer cells to thrive. It is better to use extra light olive oil, or fresh flaxseed oil.

It is best to eat grains such as barley flakes, kamut, millet, oatmeal, brown rice. By adding walnuts, bananas, and/or sorghum molasses this makes a tasty breakfast. (If you are not facing cancer, a bit of soy milk added is ok). Many of the foods just mentioned contain an ingredient known as nitriloside. As we will be see in the next chapter, nitriloside is a naturally occurring ingredient in a large number of foods that has been shown to be highly beneficial as a shield against cancer.

I often soak oatmeal in water over night. During the night, enzymes from the grain are released in the water. The next morning I pour the enzyme-rich water off the grain and drink it prior to preparing and eating the soaked grain.

For ease of digestion, it is important to consume small portions of whole foods that are tasty and naturally prepared. For the most part, they should contain their own live enzymes. Following are a few notably beneficial foods:

■ Fresh (raw) deep green (the greener the better) leafy vegetables (i.e. collard greens, mustard greens, turnip greens, kale, swiss chard, beet tops, spinach) and the fresh squeezed juices from these vegetables.

■ Garlic, and onions.

■ Green tea.

■ Turmeric, curry, basil, oregano, thyme, curcumin, and ginger root (cook with them often, especially when cooking beans, peas, and stir fries, they are high in nitriloside).

■ Broccoli sprouts, bean sprouts, alfalfa sprouts, radish sprouts. Fresh sprouts are excellent sources of protein and they contain an abundance of protein digesting enzymes. Broccoli sprouts are known to contain sulforophane, which induces the body to increase production of important detoxification enzymes.

■ Sweet potatoes, yams, lentils, brown rice, lima beans, cabbage, carrots, radishes, green peppers, celery, licorice, parsnips, cassava (yucca root), cauliflower, mint, brussel sprouts, celery, cucumbers, romaine lettuce, green and red cabbage, dandelion greens, zucchini, chinese cabbage.

■ Tomatoes and red peppers. Research has found that people with lowest levels of lycopene (a nutrient found in tomatoes and red peppers) have a 500 percent greater risk of developing pancreatic cancer than those who consume higher amounts of lycopene.

■ Blackberries, blueberries, raspberries, marion berries. Clinical tests conducted at Hollings Cancer Institute at the Medical University of South Carolina have found that these and similar deep-colored fruits contain ellagic acid, which acts as a scavenger to bind with cancer-causing chemicals such as malignin, making them inactive so that trophoblast cells cannot grow and spread.

■ Watermelons, pineapples, papayas, mangoes, honeydew melons, apples[15], grapefruit, oranges, cantaloupe, pomegranate, figs, kiwi, guava.

■ Whole grains – oatmeal and oat products, barley, flaxseed, rye, millet, brown rice.

■ Walnuts, pistachios, avocados, flaxseed, blue-green algae.

■ Wheat grass (for juicing) – The abscisic acid found in Wheat grass has been shown to help reverse the growth of malignant tumors. For further information about this uniquely valuable food, see the writings of Drs. Virginia C. Livingston and Ann Wigmore. Also, see Eydie Mae's *How I Conquered Cancer Naturally*.

■ Rejuvelac is a highly beneficial drink that happens to be easy and convenient to make and costs only pennies. This drink is made from soaking approximately one-half cup wheat berries in about eight ounces of water for twenty-four to thirty-six hours. The resulting water is known to be rich in enzymes as well as vitamins and minerals. When the water is drunk, you can refill the glass with more water, reusing the same wheat berries (which you can buy at most health food stores). You can drink the rejuvelac water all at once, or drink it throughout the day. Repeat the process for five to six mornings before starting again with a new batch of wheat berries. After the second or third morning, some of the softened wheat berries can be chewed and swallowed; they are nutritious and pleasing to the taste.

SPROUTS ALL YEAR LONG

Fresh sprouts that grow from various seeds are known to supply the highest amount of vitamins, minerals, and enzymes than any other food per unit of calorie. They nourish and strengthen the whole body, including the immune system. And the nice thing is that sprouts can be grown in 4 to 6 days, for literally pennies, right in your kitchen window (or under the kitchen sink in the case of bean sprouts). It is truly a blessing that we have available to us this highly nutritious food that practically anyone can grow, and that digests with such ease.

Whether you live on a farm, or in a high rise

apartment, here is a food that can be grown 365 days a year. This live food is loaded with enzymes, making it an excellent and tasty addition to a salad, sandwich, or veggie wrap.

For more information on growing your own sprouts, contact a local health food store. Or, contact Mumm's Sprouting Seeds located near Shellbrook, Saskatchewan (Canada). Phone (306) 747-2935, or website: www.sprouting.com/homesprouting.htm. This firm has been selling organic sprouting seeds for many years, and they offer detailed information about sprouting your own seeds.

In earlier years, people grew many of the fruits and vegetables that they ate. During World War II, citizens were encouraged to grow a "victory garden", and this was partly to help ease the commercial demand for food at a time when the country's production capability was stretched to the limit. In my view, there is something very satisfying about growing some of the food that we eat, even if it is only a small percentage of our food.

Around 1985, I made a New Year's resolution to try each day to eat something that I had personally grown or had picked from a tree or vine.

Each year I plant a garden, pick wild berries, and sprout seeds indoors. I work on the railroad on-board cross country passenger trains, and I discovered that one way to keep my New Year's resolution was by taking sprouting seeds along on the railroad. Following is an account of my "garden on the railroad"; the quote is from the book, AMTRAKing, which I authored and published in 1994:

Sometimes about four days before leaving home on a train trip I put lentil, mung beans, or alfalfa seeds in a pint jar to sprout. By the day I'm ready to hit the rails, I have sprouting plants to take along in their same jar. They continue to sprout and grow with daily rinsing with water. I eat these plants starting about the second or third day, often sharing them with others. Needless to say, fellow passengers are usually surprised that someone brought along their own "private garden". Long distance train rides can rob the body of vital nutrients. Fresh foods that are easily digested help to restore those nutrients.

---

[14]*Food, Nutrition and Prevention of Cancer: A Global Perspective.* This Report was published by the World Cancer Research Fund. (1997).

[15]Recent research on apples—The January 12, 2002 issue of *The Lancet* (a weekly journal for physicians published in London) reports on an important research finding. Recently completed by scientists from Cornell University and Seoul National University (Korea), research shows that quercetin, which is a phytochemical found in apples, has even stronger anti-cancer activity than vitamin C. See The Lancet, Vol. 359, No. 9301.

CHAPTER 8

Vitamin B-17 – A Vital Missing Link

And God said, Behold, I have given you every herb bearing seed, which is upon the face of all the earth, and every tree in which is the fruit of a tree yielding seed; to you it shall be for meat.

– GENESIS 1:29

SUMMARY:

There is a naturally occurring ingredient found in certain whole and unprocessed foods as well as in the seeds of some fruits. This ingredient, called nitriloside, is believed to be a true cancer stopper. It combines with, and destroys cancer cells, while leaving healthy cells unharmed. This ingredient also greatly enhances the effectiveness of pancreatic enzymes. Another substance, laetrile, which is made from nitriloside, was the source of controversy in the 1970s, and this chapter revisits *that controversy. Finally, there is a discussion of cancer as a chronic metabolic illness arising from dietary deficiency.*

I n centuries past, it was common for people to include in their diets the seeds of fruits. Seeds from plants are said to be an integral part of the diet in traditional cultures such as the Navajo, the Hunzas, and the Abkhazians. It has been reported that cultures such as these have never had a case of cancer in those who ate their traditional foods. Seeds are known to contain an ingredient called nitriloside or amygdalin, also called vitamin B-17. In 1952 an eminent researcher named Dr. Ernst T. Krebs, Jr. expanded upon Dr. John Beard's research. Dr. Krebs demonstrated that cancer was a deficiency disease brought on by the lack of an essential ingredient called nitriloside (also called amygdalin).

NITRILOSIDE, A PLANT INGREDIENT RIGHTFULLY AND A PROVEN VITAMIN

For thousands of years people the world over have used plants for medicinal purposes. In fact, of the most frequently used modern drugs, most have their origin in plants. It should therefore come as no surprise that nitriloside is a naturally occurring beneficial substance found in numerous plants, many of which are edible. Nitriloside is especially prevalent in the seeds of certain fruits. Dr. Krebs noted that nitriloside is not a food in the ordinary sense, and yet it is essential for good health, it dissolves in water, and is not toxic. With that observation, Dr. Krebs identified it as a vitamin, and he named it vitamin B-17.

Vitamin B-17 (or nitriloside) is sometimes referred to as laetrile. Laetrile was actually synthesized in the laboratory from nitriloside sometime in the 1950's, it is a concentrated form of nitriloside. The book *World Without Cancer* by G. Edward Griffin records the following quote from Dr. Krebs:

"Can the water-soluble non-toxic nitrilosides properly be described as food? Probably not in the strict sense of the word. They are certainly not drugs per se . . . Since the nitrilosides are neither food nor drug, they may be considered as accessory food factors. Another term for water-soluble, nontoxic accessory food factors is vitamin."

Why then have we not heard of vitamin B-17? Why is vitamin B-17 not in the text books from which our medical practitioners get their knowledge? Simply put, it is because the scientific community has not yet recognized nitriloside as a vitamin. In that regard, let us note that William Harvey[16] was at first ridiculed for advancing the belief that blood in the body was pumped by the heart and that it circulated through the body through arteries. William Jenner, when he first developed a vaccine against smallpox, was called a quack. And in the early years, authorities did not consider Isaac Newton's laws of gravity and motion as valid, even though he offered proof.

LAETRILE KILLS CANCER CELLS, LEAVING HEALTHY CELLS UNHARMED

Laetrile became controversial in the 1970s, as the Food and Drug Administration (FDA) and pharmaceutical companies advised against it on the grounds that it allegedly contained "free" hydrogen cyanide and was therefore poisonous to the body. Dr. Philip Binzel, M.D. in his book *Alive and Well* states that the scientifically proven fact is that there is no "free" hydrogen cyanide in laetrile.

Dr. Binzel notes that cancer cells contain massive amounts of an enzyme called beta-glucosidase. On the other hand, non-cancerous or healthy tissues contain only tiny traces of this enzyme. When someone who has cancer eats a seed, or for that matter any other food that contains the vitamin B-17 nutrient, the beta-glucosidase enzymes (in their cancer cells) combines with the B-17 to produce the following: two molecules of glucose, one molecule of benzaldehyde, and one molecule of hydrogen cyanide. In this chemical reaction, it is the benzaldehyde and the hydrogen cyanide that are toxic. The benzaldehyde has been shown to produce a powerfully toxic effect that kills the cancer cells (but not the healthy cells). Further, the synergistic effect of benzaldehyde and hydrogen cyanide acting together produces a considerably stronger death blow to the cancer cell. And again, laboratory proof shows that only the cancer cells are affected (and destroyed), because only they contain any significant amount of beta-glucosidase enzyme, which causes the chemical reaction to occur in the first place.

Vitamin B-17 (or nitriloside) is any of a number of water-soluble, non-poisonous, and sugary compounds found in a large number of plants, many of which are edible. Again, this highly favorable naturally occurring ingredient that we call vitamin B-17 is capable of combining with the enzyme (beta-glucosidase) from cancer cells to produce two poisonous compounds, namely, hydrogen cyanide and benzaldehyde. These two poisonous compounds then destroy cancer cells while leaving healthy cells unharmed. If there are no cancer cells in the body, no hydrogen cyanide and benzaldehyde will be formed.

Therefore, anyone who wishes to make their body an unwelcomed place for cancer will want

---

VITAMIN B-17/LAETRILE/NITRILOSIDE
When B-17/laetrile/nitriloside comes in contact with a cancer cell, it reacts with the enzyme beta-glucosidase. In turn, beta-glucosidase is only found in cancer cells in any appreciable amounts.

HYDROGEN CYANIDE, BENZALDEHYDE AND GLUCOSE
These three sustances are produced when B-17/laetrile/ nitriloside is consumed and reacts with the beta-glucosi- dase in cancer cells. Hydrogen cyanide and benzalde- hyde are both toxic to cancer cells (but not to healthy cells), and they in turn kill the cancer cells – a clinically proven fact.

to include nitriloside-rich foods in their daily diet. When nitriloside combines with the beta-glucosidase enzyme from cancer cells the result is a target-specific reaction that destroys only the cancerous cells. So the hydrogen cyanide is NOT somehow floating around freely in the vitamin B-17 and then released. It must first be manufactured as a result of the B-17 combining with beta-glucosidase, and, beta- glucosidase is found in abundance only in cancerous tumors.

What about the danger of cyanide to the rest of the body's cells? Another enzyme, rhodanese, is always present in large quantities in healthy tissues. Rhodanese has the ability to combine with cyanide and benzaldehyde to render them beneficial to the body. Luckily, cancer cells (or malignant tumors) contain no rhodanese, thus leaving the cancerous cells completely at the mercy of the two deadly poisons (hydrogen cyanide and benzaldehyde).

In his book *Beating Cancer With Nutrition*, Dr. Patrick Quillin asks this rhetorical question of nitriloside: "Could it be that a diet high in young fresh plants . . . is like having continuous non-toxic chemotherapy to kill pockets of cancer cells before they can flourish?"

Indeed, nitriloside that occurs in certain foods

is an ideal chemotherapy that delivers cyanide to the cancer cells to kill them while leaving good cells unharmed. On the other hand, compare that with conventional chemotherapy which poisons practically everything in the body! The primary effect (not the side effect, but the primary effect) of conventional chemotherapy is to poison cancerous cells AND healthy cells. In the process it weakens the immune system, making it that much easier for any remaining cancer cells to spread. Radiation treatment, while it sometimes slows the growth of tumors, has an adverse affect on the body's immune function as well.

Cancer cells contain beta-glucosidase enzyme in abundance. this enzyme combines with B-17 or Nitroloside to form: 1.) Hydrogen Cyanide (CN), 2.) Benzaldehyde, and 3.) Sugar, as indicated below. In turn, the powerfully toxic and synergistic effect of CN and Benzaldehyde kills cancer cells.

(Normal/healthy cells do not contain beta-glucosidase in any appreciable amounts.)

Normal/healthy cells produce the enzyme rhodenase, which combines with any traces of CN to produce beneficial chemistry. But cancer cells do not have rhodenase, and they cannot avoid the destructive effect of CN and Benzaldehyde.

Before the end of this century, people will probably look back at present day conventional cancer treatment and liken it to the ancient practice of drilling holes in a patient's head to permit the escape of demons.

EAT B-17 (NITRILOSIDE-RICH) FOODS DAILY

Vitamin B-17 is a crucial ingredient in many foods that are no longer eaten with regularity in the Western World. If we are serious about wiping out cancer we must correct this. Cancer does not exist in populations where there is an abundance of this nutrient in the foods that are eaten. It is unfortunate that the modern diet in the USA and other Western countries includes less and less vitamin B-17. Here are some examples of nitriloside-rich foods:

- lima beans   black eye peas   garbanzo beans pinto beans lentil black beans cassava yams
- sprouts (from broccoli seeds, alfalfa seeds, mung beans, radish seeds; including many other sprouting seeds as well, but especially these, if you have cancer) Brewer's Yeast
- apricot kernels   peach kernels   pear seeds apple seeds   plum kernels   cherry kernels

- barley   millet   oat grain   brown rice
  brewer's yeast   sorghum molasses
- blackberries   huckleberries   raspberries
  strawberries   current   papaya
  blueberries
- goose berries   loganberries   cranberries
  boysenberries   wild crabapple   mulberries
- wheat grass   johnson grass   bermuda grass
  beet tops   bamboo shoots   Spinach
- pecans   macadamia nuts   flax seed
  walnuts   bitter almond   cashews

Some foods are higher in vitamin B-17 than others. Of the foods listed above, apricot kernels are known to contain the highest amount of B-17. Crack open the hard shell of an apricot seed and there you will find the kernal, which looks like a small almond nut. Note also, that the previous list is only a partial listing of foods that contain nitriloside.

As for a general guideline regarding dosage of B-17, Dr. Krebs suggested a minimum of fifty milligrams of B-17 daily for a normal healthy adult. Naturally, someone predisposed to cancer or already suffering from it would require much more. The average apricot kernel contains approximately 4 to 5 milligrams of B-17, but this amount can vary by as much as a factor of six. I know of healthy people who take 100 to 200 milligrams of B-17 pills. I have read of cancer patients who ate twenty or more apricot kernels daily and achieved good results.

HYDROGEN CYANIDE ENHANCES ENZYME ACTION

Nitriloside represents a potent means of not only selectively destroying cancer cells and preventing cancer, but equally important, the hydrogen cyanide (which the nitriloside helps to produce) has been shown to reactivate and accelerate the effectiveness of various pancreatic enzymes. This is a tremendous benefit because it means the hydrogen cyanide makes trypsin, chymotrypsin, amylase and lipase work even better!

HOW MUCH B-17 IS ENOUGH?

How can we determine if there is a sufficient level of B-17 (or nitriloside) in the body? It turns out that nitrilosides can be monitored, because when the body metabolizes nitrilosides, the by product is something called thiocyanate. Dr. Binzel notes in his book *Alive and Well* that thiocyanate levels in the blood can be measured. He indicates that patients who do best are those that maintain between 1.2 and 2.5 milligrams of thiocyanate per decaliter of blood. Of course, the desired amount of thiocyanate in the blood is a matter for health care professionals to determine depending on the individual patient.

LAETRILE IS BANNED

As we already mentioned, during the 1970s vitamin B-17 (also called laetrile) was discredited vigorously by the American medical community, the pharmaceutical industry, and the FDA. Laetrile was eventually banned by the FDA. However, cancer patients who were said to be "terminally ill" often petitioned the courts and were granted permission to import laetrile from Mexico. At the same time, distinguished physicians in various parts of the world were getting good results with laetrile and they strongly advocated its use. Unfortunately, most people were not aware of these and other physicians who were obtaining successful results from laetrile treatment of cancer.

There has been very little written about B-17 and its benefits in the last twenty-five years. But we should not let that cause us to hastily conclude that this vital substance is unimportant. Dr. Kanematsu Sugiura was on the staff at the Memorial Sloan Kettering Institute in the 1970s as a cancer biochemist.

He was arguably America's leading cancer biochemist in those years, and he performed studies on B-17 (or laetrile). He found that it caused complete tumor regression in some laboratory mice and partial regression in others. Unfortunately, however, Sloan-Kettering announced that the results of Dr. Sugiura's research were not significant, and thus chose not to extend the research to humans.

This leading cancer research facility then proceeded to suppress the part of his work that showed that nitriloside eliminated or reduced tumors in laboratory animals. Eventually, however, individuals within Sloan-Kettering "leaked" the report to the outside world.[17]

FAMOUS PHYSICIANS WHO HAVE SUPPORTED B-17 WITH GOOD RESULTS

Dr. Hans Nieper is former director of the Department of Medicine at Silbersee Hospital in Hanover, Germany. He is also the former director of the German Society for Medical Tumour Treatment, and is listed in Who's Who in the World of Science. During a visit to the USA in 1972, Dr. Nieper told reporters:

"After more than twenty years of such specialized work, I have found non-toxic nitrilosides – that is, laetrile – are superior to any other known cancer treatment or preventative. In my opinion, it is the only existing possibility for the ultimate control of cancer."

Dr. N.R. Bouziane is the former Director of Research Laboratories at St. Jeanne D'Arc Hospital in Montreal, Canada. He received a doctorate degree in science from the University of Montreal. Dr. Bouziane's repeated success in treating cancers with laetrile were written up in the *Cancer News Journal*, January/April 1971, p.20, under the article titled "The Laetrile Story".

Dr. Manual Navarro is a former Professor of Medicine and Surgery in Manila, the Philippines. He held many prestigious titles in the field of science and is an internationally recognized cancer researcher with over one hundred major scientific papers to his credit, some of which were presented before the International Cancer Congress. Dr. Navarro stated in the *Cancer News Journal*:

"It is my carefully considered clinical judgement as a practicing oncologist and researcher in this field, that I have obtained most significant encouraging results with the use of laetrile – amygdalin in the treatment of terminal cancer patients . . ."

An Italian medical school professor named Dr. Etore Guidetti addressed the Conference of the International Union Against Cancer held in Brazil in 1954, and announced startling results with laetrile successfully combating many types of cancers.[18]

In the USA a number of respected and highly distinguished physicians and scientists embraced laetrile from the 1950s to the 1970s when it was banned in the USA. Some of the physicians and researchers in the USA include Dr. Ernst T. Krebs, Jr., who developed laetrile, Dr. Harold Mann, professor of biology at Loyola University in Chicago, Dr. H. Ray Ever, Dr. John A. Richardson of Albany New York, and Dr. Dean Burk, to name a few. Dr. Burk was a founding member of the American National Cancer Institute, he was the recipient of several prestigious awards in the field, and he published over two hundred scientific papers in the field of cell chemistry, and authored three books on cancer research.[19]

From the 1980s and on, laetrile has rarely been a topic of discussion in health and medical publications or in the media in general. Nevertheless, there is undeniable evidence that foods rich in nitriloside are vital to both cancer prevention and cancer cure. And remember that nitriloside is the naturally occurring ingredient found in various fruits and vegetables from which laetrile is made.

Fortunately, you and I do not have to go hunting for laetrile or amygdalin, which are basically the laboratory forms of vitamin B17. We do not have to reinvent the 1970's controversy. We simply have to include in our daily diet foods that already have naturally occurring nitriloside as an ingredient.

CANCER AND DIETARY DEFICIENCY

Not many people nowadays know much about the following diseases: scurvy, rickets, pellagra, beri beri, night blindness, and pernicious anemia. These are vitamin deficiency diseases that killed millions of people beginning in the Middle Ages and into the 1900's when the medical industry started accepting the idea that these chronic metabolic illnesses could be eliminated with food substances called vitamins.

It turns out that deficiencies in vitamins C, B3, A, B12, D and B1 proved to be the answer. But widespread use of these vitamins was delayed for many years after their original discovery because medical practice was slow to accept the idea that satisfying a dietary deficiency could hold the key to curing these diseases. As a result, in the years immediately following the discovery of the vitamins, many people continued to die needlessly.

Even as late as 1900 many doctors still held to the Louis Pasteur doctrine of the 1860s that most diseases were infectious and caused by microscopic organisms. Doctors were less inclined to see some illnesses as being related to diet and metabolism. As a result, people died simply because they were ignorant of the facts. British sailors died by the tens of thousands from scurvy during the eighteenth and nineteenth centuries.

In 1753, Scottish naval surgeon James Land discovered that an unknown nutrient (vitamin C) in citrus fruits prevented scurvy. Unfortunately, his findings were largely ignored for about forty years during which time British sailors continued to die needlessly. Eventually, everyone got the message that vitamin C was the answer to scurvy. With rickets, for instance, prevention was eventually found to be as simple as increasing exposure to sunlight, and including vitamin D in the diet.

As early as 1914 Dr. Joseph Goldberger demonstrated that the disease pellagra was caused by nutritional deficiency, and he even showed that it could be prevented by eating liver or yeast. But not until the 1940s was it conceded by the medical establishment that pellagra was indeed a vitamin B deficiency. Today, if you ask the average person what is scurvy, rickets, and pellagra, many could not give a correct answer because those diseases have all but been eliminated.

Remember, these are all chronic metabolic-related diseases, they did not come about from germs. A chronic illness is one that does not go away on its own; and a metabolic illness is one that occurs within the body and cannot be transmitted to another person. Cancer is also a chronic metabolic illness. It is not a disease that spreads due to some germ or virus. And just as diet and nutrition were eventually accepted as the answer to scurvy, rickets, pellagra, and other chronic metabolic diseases, we therefore would do well to look more carefully at diet and nutrition as the major answer to cancer. Regrettably, our society

VITAMIN DEFICIENCY DISEASES

Recorded history shows that all of the diet-deficiency diseases listed here and their corresponding cures had to overcome strong and long-lasting resistance from the established medical community. With each of these diseases, the cause was nutritional deficiency, and the cure was the reversal of that deficiency.

Disease	Vitamin to alleviate this disease
Scurvy	C
Pellagra	B3
Night Blindness	A
Pernicious Anemia	B12
Rickets	D
Beri Beri	B1
Cancer	**B-17 (The Missing Link?)**

It seems clear that the final resolution of cancer (also an illness that derives from a diet deficiency) depends not on a new chemical compound with its inevitable drug effects, but on a dietary regimen that will reverse the deficiency.

---

in large part has yet to respond with commitment to cancer as a metabolic illness that relates to a dietary deficiency.

Think about this for a moment: each of the diseases mentioned above were caused not by something that people did, but by something they did not do. That is, people did not include in their diets the various vitamins we have been discussing. We typically think of a disease like cancer as being caused by something we did, such as smoking cigarettes, eating refined and fatty foods, drinking polluted water, breathing polluted air, too much stress, etc. We do not generally consider that cancer might be caused by something we did not do, or did not eat.

Admittedly, there is evidence that risk factors such as smoking cigarettes, poor diet, and poor water and air quality and stress all play an important role. However, I submit that we miss an opportunity to get to the root of cancer when we fail to consider that this devastating illness arises in large part because of our failure to include more nitriloside-rich foods in our daily diet.

In truth, no chronic metabolic disease has ever found real cure or real prevention except through factors essential to diet and lifestyle. There is extensive evidence to indicate that the incidence, severity, and control of cancer depends more on diet than any other single factor, with nitriloside-rich foods as a priority.

We should in all fairness note that the National Cancer Institute, and mainstream medical personnel in general acknowledge the importance of diet as a preventative measure against cancer. Doctors routinely counsel their patients to "eat your broccoli," "cut down on fatty foods," and "eat fresh fruit". In addition, the American Cancer Society has prepared extensive guidelines on nutrition for anyone concerned about cancer. The first guideline listed is: "eat a variety of healthful foods, with an emphasis on plant sources."

This concern for diet and nutrition is strongly promoted by many health care professionals, especially as long as the issue is cancer prevention. But if cancer is ever discovered in someone, most people at that point (healthcare professionals included) then consider the issue of diet and nutrition to be too little too late. Instead, they opt for drugs, and medical procedures that all too often place the patient's overall health at even greater risk, while sometimes controlling the cancer but never curing it.

We saw how with scurvy, rickets, pellagra and other metabolic diseases it took many years from when the particular vitamin deficiency was first identified to when medical practice routinely accepted the vitamin (or food substance) as the cure. Similarly, it may require many more years before established medical practitioners and lay people alike start looking seriously to diet as a major factor in recovering from cancer.

The best news of all is that you and I do NOT have to wait for the medical community to come aboard this train!

G. Edward Griffin notes in his book *World Without Cancer* the successful experiences of numerous people who started and maintained a diet rich in vitamin B-17 foods. He states that:

"For over two decades there has been a steadily growing group of people who have accepted the vitamin theory of cancer who have altered their diets accordingly. They represent all walks of life, all ages, both sexes, and reside in almost every advanced nation of the world. It is estimated that there are many thousands in the United States alone. It is significant, therefore, that after starting and maintaining a diet rich in vitamin B-17 (nitriloside), none of these people have ever been known to contract cancer."

The famous medical missionary, Dr. Albert Schweitzer, once noted the absence of cancer in connection with a trip that he made to West Africa. He said: "On my arrival in Gabon in 1913, I was astonished to encounter no cases of cancer. I saw none among the natives two hundred miles from the coast . . . this absence of cancer seemed to be due to the difference in the nutrition of the natives compared to the Europeans . . ." Cassava is a food that has traditionally been consumed in abundance in West Africa, and cassava has a high content of naturally occurring nitriloside.

It's Not enough to Simply Avoid Meat and Dairy

Readers should be aware that merely abstaining from animal protein and pasteurized dairy is not sufficient if they want to minimize the risk of cancer. What is more important is that the daily diet include fresh uncooked fruits, vegetables, and nuts, and especially foods that have nitriloside. As has been emphasized, fresh foods have their own enzymes to facilitate their digestion, and they often have extra enzymes that can combine with and dissolve the protein/starchy coating from around cancer cells that otherwise "hides" the cancer cells from the immune system.

We are well advised to eat more complex carbohydrates such as yams, sweet potatoes, lentil, lima beans, black beans, squash, avocados, and foods made from whole grains. These and other nitriloside-rich foods like fresh blueberries, black-berries, raspberries, black-eye peas, brown rice, turmeric spice and leafy green vegetables are very powerful guardians that fortify the body against cancer when eaten daily.

It is possible to state with a high degree of certainty that increased cancer rates derive more from the fact that we are NOT eating enough nitriloside-rich foods, and less from the fact that we indulge in unhealthful practices like tobacco usage and high meat consumption. Please do not misunderstand me, these unhealthful practices are definite risk factors. But one can successfully argue that the inclusion of lots of nitriloside foods in the daily diet reduces the cancer risk and less-ens the adverse affects of otherwise unhealthful practices.

Eskimos have traditionally eaten a high meat diet, but they do not get cancer. Much of the meat they eat is from caribou animals that graze on the range eating grass high in nitriloside. That is not the case, however, with commercially grown beef cattle, as they are raised in feed lots where the ani-mals are fed not grass but grain that contains very little if any nitriloside.

Also, some ethnic groups in Africa eat meat

and they don't get cancer. Again, they eat animals that graze on nitriloside-rich grass. They also eat a lot of plants that contain nitriloside. It is true that they contract other illnesses, but not cancer. Parts of India and surrounding countries have very low incidence of cancer. Again, they contract other illnesses, but not cancer. The people in these places include in their daily diets spices like turmeric and curry, and lots of green vegetables – all high in nitriloside.

More than twenty-five years ago pharmaceutical companies and the medical establishment pushed the FDA into making it illegal to sell "raw" apricot seeds (the richest known source of nitrilosides or vitamin B-17) as a cure for cancer. To this day, it is difficult to find apricot kernels at most health food stores. As of this writing, one of the few sources to acquire this food is American Biologics in Chula Vista, California. They sell a one-pound package of organically grown and sundried (not roasted) apricot kernels for approximately $14. You can reach them at 1-800-227-4473, or see www.americanbiologics.com.

Still not convinced that B-17 (nitriloside rich) foods are cancer stoppers? Be sure to read Phillip Day's book, *Cancer: Why We're Still Dying To Know*

The Truth, copyright 2001, ISBN 0953501248; especially see pages 110 - 114 of his well-researched work.

Still not convinced that B-17(nitriloside-rich)
foods are cancer stoppers? Be sure to read Phillip
Day's book, *Cancer: Why We're Still Dying To Know
The Truth,* copyright 2001, ISBN 0953501248; especially see pages 110-114 of his well-researched work.
In addition, Mr. Day notes at pages 42-57 that several attempts have been made to present "victims"
of apricot seed poisoning to the public in an attempt
to discredit B-17, but that these attempts have all
been exposed as frauds. He demonstrates that physicians and researchers who support B-17 therapy
vigorously endorse this vitamin's harmlessness
when used within researched guidelines.

*"And God said, Behold, I have given you every herb
bearing seed . . . to you it shall be for meat.*

– Genesis 1:29

---

[16]William Harvey is credited with having been the first to expound the
theory that blood circulates in our veins and is pumped by the heart.

[17]See G. Edward Griffin's book *World Without Cancer* (ISBN: 0-912986-19-0).
His is a well documented and often quoted work first published in 1974,
with fourteen reprints by 1998. Also, see Chapter 2 of Maureen Salaman's
Nutrition: The Cancer Answer (1996).

[18]Information from this paragraph and the paragraphs immediately
preceding is from an article "The Politics of Death" from the United
Kingdom publication titled *Credence Publications.*
See: www.credence.org/doctors.html. Also, there are approximately 35
pages of testimonials describing the successful results of laetrile.
See: www.credence.org/testimon.html.

[19]See: Cancer News Journal. January/April 1971.

An Answer to Cancer's Wake Up Call

"Each patient carries his own doctor inside him.
They come to us not knowing that truth.
We are at our best when we give the doctor who
resides in each patient a chance to go to work."

Dr. Albert Schweitzer

I believe deeply in the body's ability to heal it-self of a metabolic diet deficiency illness if given the right opportunity. **If I personally am ever suspected of having cancer, the following are some thoughts I would embrace, and things I would do immediately; many of them I already do as a matter of routine:**

■ I will stop eating animal products – no beef, pork, chicken, etc., except for an occasional serving of salmon – and no eggs nor pasteurized dairy products.

■ Will drink four ounces, four times a day of fresh squeezed vegetable juice made from deep green leafy vegetables such as collard greens, turnip and mustard greens, kale greens, or bok choy, and I'll mix this juice with fresh squeezed carrot and celery juice. If it is possible to get it, I will alternate some days and drink fresh juice from wheat grass. Also, I will add fresh ginger to these drinks to get the benefit of its cooling effects.

■ Will eat pineapple, papaya and figs, and will juice these fruits daily in order to introduce vitally important protein digesting enzymes into my body. I will juice the outside covering of the pineapple as well, processing it in a slow rpm juicer in order to derive maximum benefit from its bromelain enzyme.

■ Will consume roughly 75 percent raw fruits and vegetables. The main fruits will be watermelons, pineapples, papayas, mangoes, grapefruits, blackberries, raspberries, and blueberries. In addition to assorted deep green leafy vegetables. I will eat a handful of sprouts (especially broccoli sprouts) daily. I will also eat yams, black-eyed peas, lima beans, lentils, brown rice, tomatoes, and spices such as garlic, turmeric, curry, and oregano.

■ Will eat ten to twenty apricot kernels daily, chewing them thoroughly. I will also consume each day other foods that contain vitamin B-17 (or nitriloside) to include lentils, lima beans, brown rice, millet, flaxseed meal, sorghum molasses, wheat grass, bean sprouts, yucca root, and wild berries such as raspberries, blackberries, and blueberries.

■ Will obtain protein mainly from avocados, sprouts, blue-green algae and occasional small amounts of nuts such as almonds, walnuts, pecans, pistachios. I will eat no protein foods after 1 p.m. daily because cancer challenges the body's ability to digest protein, any protein. This allows roughly eighteen hours a day for the body to generate protein digesting enzymes that are so vital for dissolving the protein/starchy coating from around the cancer cells.

■ Will purchase a good digestive enzyme supple-

ment (in powdered form) and use it daily, sprin-
kling it on lunch and dinner foods that are cooked.
I will make a point of chewing my food thoroughly, and never over eating or stuffing
myself.

■ Will drink green tea extract, three to four cups
daily. The chlorophyll in green tea contains magnesium, which is vital for carrying oxygen to all
parts of the body. The increased abundance of oxygen in turn suppresses tumor growth. Another
ingredient in green tea is known to help break
down malignant tumor masses. Also, the hot
water in green tea helps flush out toxins.

■ Will exercise daily for half an hour-by walking, swimming, bicycling, working in the garden,
or using the trampoline or stationary cycle. These
and other aerobic activities distribute oxygen to
all parts of the body, and they exercise the vitally
important lymph system. An oxygen-rich body
helps to suppress tumor growth, since cancerous
cells do not thrive in oxygen. I will also do deep
breathing often, as this too distributes more oxygen to body tissues. (I am a blues harmonica
player, and luckily, I automatically do a lot of deep

breathing while playing this delightful little instrument).

■ Will do something each day to achieve a feeling of peace of mind and wholeness – walking in nature, listening to soothing music, expressing thanks to God for little things, playing old time favorites like "Danny Boy" and "Amazing Grace" on my harmonica.

■ Will avoid getting a biopsy or CAT scan, and instead will choose less invasive and less health compromising procedures, such as MRI tests, blood tests, cancer marker tests, and chorionic gonadotropic (CGH) tests. Biopsies and CAT scans accurately pinpoint the malignancy and give detailed information about the chemistry of the tumor, but they do so at great risk to the underlying health of the patient, thus presenting an added challenge to an already overburdened immune system. For me, it is less important to know the exact size, location, and chemistry of the tumor mass; what is far more important is whether cancer exists, and if it does I intend to attack it aggressively through diet and lifestyle changes. Neither biopsies nor CAT scans are to be taken lightly. Biopsies are minor surgical procedures that disturb the tumor mass, create scar tissue, and increase the possibility of the tumor spreading. CAT scans require that chemicals be injected into the body, chemicals that add an extra burden to an already challenged liver. Admittedly, biopsies, and perhaps CAT scans would be a medical requirement for almost anyone who plans to go for chemotherapy, radiation, or surgery. But I do not anticipate subjecting my body to such procedures.

■ I will eliminate white flour, white sugar, most commercial oils, honey and most other sugary syrups except sorghum molasses. Concentrated refined sugar (which the body digests as glucose) and simple carbohydrates (which the body converts to glucose) are the two primary foods from which cancerous cell masses derive their energy to live and grow. As we saw in chapter 2, cancer cells manufacture their energy from glucose alone, without oxygen; so it is vitally important to deny them this essential source of their energy. Additionally, I will avoid eating peanuts, since they contain a protein that happens to be difficult for cancer patients to digest. A scientific study by professor George Bailey at Oregon State University indicates that peanuts can carry a toxic substance called aflatoxin that has been shown to be cancer-causing.

■ Will drink a cup of fresh squeezed beet juice twice a week, for the purpose of cleansing my liver. This is important because the liver filters the toxic tumor tissue that is being broken down and which the body is trying to expel.

■ Will take one tablespoon of fresh cod liver oil 3 to 4 times a week. It is one of the best sources of the essential fatty acid Omega 3 (which our bodies often lack), yet is so vital for good health.

■ Will drink at least eight glasses of water daily (non-chlorinated if possible), and will try to avoid exposure to the toxic chemicals found in most commercial cleaners. All functions of the body are regulated by the flow of water. Without water, for instance, the body could not dissolve the oxygen that it so urgently needs for suppressing cancer cells and revitalizing good cells. I will drink several swallows of water prior to eating a meal, as it is beneficial to the initiation of the digestion process. Without water, cell activity diminishes. Water also improves bowel transit time and facilitates internal cleansing. According to Dr. Batmanghelidj, water prevents the body from producing excessive histamine, and too much histamine suppresses the immune system.

■ I will drink rejuvelac daily. To make it, just put one cup of spring wheat and three cups of water in a container and let it sit for twenty-four hours; then pour off the water and drink it throughout the day. Repeat this for up to six days; then start with a new batch of wheat berries. This high quality, fermented drink is loaded with enzymes that facilitate digestion, and it also helps maintain intestinal flora in the small intestine. In addition, this simple and very inexpensive drink is high in vitamins E and K and in pre-digested sugars and amino acids. Wheat berries can be purchased inexpensively at most health food stores. (For more information about rejuvelac, see Eydie Mae's *How I Conquered Cancer*, 1992.

■ Will spend time in a sauna once or twice a week. Heat helps remove excess acidity from the body, and tests have shown that cancerous cells have difficulty surviving in temperatures that are seven or eight degrees higher than normal body temperature.

■ Will make an effort to expose myself to direct sunlight at least an hour a day. This is crucial for synthesizing vitamin D. Being of African ancestry, I happen to have dark skin. To insure that adequate vitamin D is synthesized in my body, I require exposure to more sunlight than someone who is of fair complexion or whose skin is without pigment. Vitamin D synthesized from natural sunlight is far superior to vitamin D dietary supplements. Studies have linked deficiencies in this vitamin with cancer.

■ I will consult with competent health care professionals whose medical practice focuses mainly on the enzyme treatment of cancer.

Many readers will say that the points just mentioned represent extreme action. They are right!

When cancer arises, you must take extreme action, you "call the cops"! At a minimum, you must immediately start doing moderate physical exercise and deep breathing in order to oxygenate the body tissue, take fresh squeezed green vegetable juice (four ounces four times a day) , eat raw vegetables, avoid meat and other animal products as well as white sugar and white flour, and drink at least eight glasses of water a day. Personally, I prefer to "call 911" for these "natural health cops", as opposed to other "cops" that bring with them poisonous chemicals and knife blades.

It is very important to understand that at the cellular level, the basis for any cancer has to do with several factors, and they include:

1. The body's inability to manufacture enough of certain enzymes that digest proteins.

2. Insufficient oxygen circulating throughout the body.

3. A weak immune system that is unable to target cancer cells and destroy them.

4. Overall body chemistry that is highly acidic (and thus conducive to tumor growth).

In addition, cancer is able to emerge when someone has a dietary deficiency from not eating enough fresh fruits, vegetables, and nuts that contain vitamin B-17 (nitriloside).

But all is not lost. Instead, each of us can do something about cancer merely by the way we nourish our physical bodies and go about our daily lives.

What a blessing to know that, given the right focus and commitment, we as individuals can make a difference in preventing and overcoming this dreaded illness.

CHAPTER 10 —————————————————

Recipe Suggestions

Here are a few good tasting food choices. In addition to providing vitamins and minerals, they nourish the body by fostering a cellular environment rich in oxygen, alkaline in chemistry, and they introduce important enzymes.

Here is a recipe for my favorite Tahini Salad Dressing, a tasty complement to deep green leafy vegetables:

1/4 cup of fresh squeezed lemon juice
1/2 cup oil (flaxseed oil or extra light olive oil)
1/4 cup tamari
1/3 cup tahini
1/8 cup of water
2 finely chopped garlic cloves
1 tablespoon sorghum molasses

Here is a recipe for a delicious yams (or sweet potato) stir fry:

Dice yams (or sweet potatoes) for frying
Chop up some onions, garlic, and fresh ginger root
Fry all of the above ingredients using safflower or olive oil. While cooking, add a teaspoon of tumeric and a teaspoon of curry spices. Stir often to insure the potatoes get cooked, and when they are done this dish is ready for eating.

Optional: just before the yams are cooked, throw in some fresh or frozen green peas.

Try this tasty dish as part of your lunch or dinner:

One cup of dry lima beans — soak them in water for 12 to 24 hours. Pour off the water. (Feel free to drink some of this water, since it is rich in enzymes from the soaked beans).

Next, put fresh water into the pot of soaked beans, filling it about one inch beyond the height of the beans. Let this cook very slowly for about an hour, then add one-half cup chopped onions and 1/2 cup chopped ginger root. Now add 2 teaspoons of tumeric, one teaspoon of curry, a teaspoon of sorghum molasses and a teaspoon of tamari sauce.

Let the ingredients continue cooking very slowly for another two hours or more until done. About one-half hour before it is done, I sometimes add a chopped carrot, and a hand full of chopped cabbage.

Note: It is advisable (especially if someone has cancer) to take a digestive aid such as pancreatin (preferably in powder form) along with this meal. It will facilitate digestion, since the cooked beans and vegetables have no enzymes. Be sure to eat a serving of uncooked deep green leafy vegetables as a salad everyday with lunch and dinner, and always include some of those enzyme and nutrient-rich sprouts in every salad – they can be grown easily right under the kitchen sink!

One can prepare black beans, black eye peas, pinto beans, and others in a similar way as lima beans to make a tasty and nutritious dish filled with nitriloside-rich foods.

A Tasty Corn Tortilla

1 corn tortilla – lightly heated in a plain skillet
Add: generous slices of avocado, tomatoes, and chopped greens (collards, turnip, mustard, spinach, kale)
Pour on tahini salad dressing (from recipe shown previously)
Fold the tortilla, and prepare for delicious eating. At other times, add some brown rice to the vegetable mix.

Try this Scrumptious Fruit Pie

To make a single crust:

Mix together one-half cup of ground flaxseed meal, 3/4 cup of whole wheat flour, 1 cup of oatmeal flour, 1/2 teaspoon of sea salt. Stir these ingredients well, and gradually add one-half cup of extra light olive oil. Cut in the olive oil with a fork or pastry blender until the dough is like cornmeal in thickness or like small peas. Now, sprinkle on four to five tablespoons of cold water, all while gently stirring the dough into a ball. Flatten the dough on a lightly floured surface, and roll it out with a rolling pin to form a pie crust. Transfer the crust into a nine-inch pie plate and cook it in the oven at 375 degrees for 12 to 15 minutes.

Adding the fruit to the crust:

When the crust is done and has cooled, pour fresh black berries, blue berries, peaches, etc into it. If fresh fruit is not available, use frozen fruit that has been allowed to thaw out on its own. Sprinkle on a few shakes of nutmeg, and squeeze a few twists of lemon juice over the fruit. Finally, pour roughly two tablespoons of sorghum molasses over the fruit. The pie is now ready to eat.

BREAKFAST SUGGESTIONS

Fresh Fruit – Especially deep purple berries, papaya, figs, pineapple, bananas, grapefruit, oranges.

Whole grains – Oatmeal, barley, ground flaxseed, brown rice, whole wheat.

Soy Milk – Use sparingly, as it is high in protein and since it (like cooked meat) is without enzymes, it therefore competes with the malignant tumor for pancreatic digestive enzymes. Raw goat milk is better.

Nuts – Almonds, pecans, walnuts (The fresher the better. Soak them overnight in water, and/or be sure to chew them thoroughly to release their enzyme inhibitors to facilitate their digestion).

Sorghum molasses – Good as an occasional syrup on whole grain pancakes.

Generally, someone facing cancer should consider eating fruits, vegetables, nuts and seeds along with complex carbohydrates like lima beans, black beans, black eye peas, squash, yams, brown rice and avocados. They should season their complex carbohydrates with spices like tumeric, curry, ginger root, onions and garlic. Except for breakfast, grains, even whole grains, should be a minor part of the diet.

Also, except for breakfast, every meal should include a generous serving of fresh uncooked deep green leafy vegetables to always include fresh sprouts, and a portion of avocado. This salad should always be the centerpiece of the meal. Feel free to use the tasty tahini salad dressing whose recipe is shown on page 119. Drinks should mainly include water, and herb tea, especially green tea. Between meal snacks – fresh fruit, a few nuts (before mid day), raw vegetables.

Again, if someone has cancer, a highly important thing to include in their daily eating regimen is four ounces of fresh squeezed deep green vegetable juice four times a day, consumed preferably on an empty stomach or between meals. Anyone who has read previous chapters of this book will undoubtedly understand the importance of this.

Also, see *The Little Cyanide Cookbook: Delicious Recipes Rich in Vitamin B-17* by June de Spain. See www.realityzone.com, then click on "health issues".

FIRST LINE OF DEFENSE
AGAINST CANCER

Eat foods (especially raw foods) that contain digestive enzymes similar to the enzymes secreted by the pancreas. Certain enzymes are capable of dissolving the protein and starchy coating from around cancer cells, and this exposes the cancer cells to the immune system which can then target them for destruction. The following foods are especially beneficial in this regard: papaya, pineapple, deep green leafy vegetables, avocados, wheat grass juice, broccoli sprouts, and fruits and vegetables with deep committed colors.

SECOND LINE OF DEFENSE
AGAINST CANCER

Eat foods that contain nitriloside. Nitriloside is a naturally occuring substance in dozens of foods – to include lentils, lima beans, brown rice, green leafy vegetables, blackberries, raspberries, blueberries, turmeric and ginger, to mention a few. If there are cancerous cells in the body, the nitriloside in the food combines with an enzyme that's found only in the cancer cells and it produces substances that are toxic only to the cancer cells, thus destroying them. Foods with the highest content of nitriloside are seeds from fruits – especially apricot kernels.

IN SUMMARY

■ **Oxygenate the body tissues** – Exercise; breathe deeply; eat chlorophyll rich foods (i.e., green foods), they contain magnesium which carries oxygen throughout the body. Oxygen greatly enhances healthy tissues, while it suppresses cancerous tissues. See chapter 2 for details.

■ **Drink water** – Make a conscious effort to drink at least 8 glasses of water daily. Water, and water alone, is essential to the proper functioning of every cell in the body. Drink a cup of water about one-half hour before meals to facilitate digestion of the meal. Drink water approximately two hours following a meal. Try it, it works!

■ Build a strong immune system – The body's overall immune function will destroy cancer cells provided it is able to "see" and recognize them, and provided the immune system is strong and vibrant.

■ Enzymes are key – Eat live foods, as they are abundant with enzymes. Certain enzymes will dissolve the protein and starchy substance that covers cancer cells and that otherwise hides them from the immune system. The enzymes trypsin, chymotrypsin, amylase, and lipase are the body's first shield of protection against cancer. They are the sine qua non for cancer resolution. Don't be caught without them!

■ Nitrilosides – Eat foods daily that contain these little-talked-about but highly valuable food ingredients. Nitrilosides perform a kind of ongoing and natural chemotherapy function by killing cancer cells that escaped the immune system's policing action. (And unlike conventional chemotherapy, nitrilosides do not kill healthy cells). Take heed, nitrilosides are the body's second shield of protection against cancer. Learn the foods that contain nitrilosides and eat some with every meal.

In sum, it is entirely possible for someone to maintain a shield of protection against cancer: exercise regularly to create oxygen-rich body tissues, eat foods that result in an overall alkaline body chemistry, eat green foods, enzyme-rich foods, and nitriloside-rich foods. As we have seen, they go to work right away at the cellular level to check the growth of cancerous tissue; and best of all, they can do it without creating unfavorable "side effects" such as impairing the immune system.

There is compelling evidence to suggest that the illness we call cancer is a direct outgrowth of our modern life in the Western World. Directly implicated is the stressful lives that we often lead, the chemicals in our drinking water, lack of physical exercise, chemicals in our food, the polluted air we breathe, and even the chemicals we breathe in our kitchens and bathrooms. Add to that the fact that an incredibly high percentage of our food consists of animal products, and cooked, refined and processed foods. The typical Western diet involves only a hint of deep green leafy vegetables, fresh fruits, and nuts. The combined effect of all this is to make our body chemistry highly acidic and lacking in oxygen at the cellular level. It's in this environment that malignant tumor cells are able to thrive.

To be sure, diet is not the only factor in our modern way of life that has an impact on cancer. But it is the one important factor that we each can influence moment to moment.

As we have discussed throughout this book, cancer manifests as malignant tumors in various parts of the body – whether they be in the breast, colon, prostate, pancreas, liver, brain, etc. But the underlying cause of any malignant tumor is associated with a cellular environment that is invariably oxygen- starved, often water-starved, over acidic, and deficient in certain pancreatic enzymes.

As we know, the standard response to cancer is to try and eliminate the symptom, that is, the malignant tumor either by chemotherapy, radiation, or surgery – all with little regard for their adverse affects on the immune system and the body's overall health. Unfortunately, there is little focus on the cancer, that is, on the process that caused the malignant tumor in the first place. Often the malignant tumor is removed, yet the patient goes on doing more or less the things that caused the tumor in the first place. Visit the cancer ward of most hospitals today and you will often find patients eating meat, cheese, simple sugars and starches, and refined and processed foods.

One thing is clear: cancer cannot gain a foothold in a body where there are sufficient protein digesting enzymes, where tissues are well oxygenated, and where the blood and the small intestine maintain an alkaline pH without stealing from other parts of the body.

Clearly, a major component to the answer to cancer lies not in yet another miracle drug to suppress symptoms, but in a fundamental change in the way we live. It means we have to respect the sanctity of our body, and take greater personal responsibility for it's physical and spiritual nourishment.

A Spiritual Perspective

"Everything has been figured out,
except how to live."

JEAN-PAUL SARTRE

Cancer cries out for us to do more than treat it's symptom. It is important that we approach it holistically. In that regard, there is a spiritual component that must always influence our attitude and support all that we do in seeking to either prevent or recover from cancer. Cancer challenges us to look beyond our human selves and connect with the Christ Spirit within us.

Dr. William D. Kelley is a dentist who in 1965 cured himself of advanced pancreatic cancer. As of this writing, Dr. Kelley is still living and remains cancer free. He documented his recovery experiences in the book *"One Answer to Cancer"*, copyright 1998, ISBN 09669422-0-5. Chapter VII of his book begins as follows:

"If your cancer has caused you to stop, think, pray, and know God better, it has been a blessing to you.

If your cancer has caused you to realize the importance and magnificence of this temple wherein your soul dwells, you have been doubly blessed."

Regardless of your physical condition, if you want to change your body, change your awareness. Commune with the Creator often through prayer and meditation, and KNOW in your heart that the Christ Spirit within you has perfect health. That level of awareness is all that is needed in order to proceed with confidence to visualize your body as being free of sickness.

Have faith in God, and KNOW that God will never leave you. Faith replaces fear and anxiety with the peace and joy for living each day – and living not as a "cancer fighter", but as a Child of God who welcomes each day's gifts, even while facing the challenge of a serious illness.

The apostle Paul counseled his fellow churchmen to "...pray without ceasing." It's important that we pray for divine guidance and for the determination to stick with a protocol that brings healing to the underlying cause of cancer. Pray for the wisdom to understand God's will. Through

prayer, God is revealed to us as a Higher Presence
that protects and is as close to us as our very own
breath. My grandmother in Fargo, Arkansas used
to sing a soulful refrain, it was titled What A
Friend We Have In Jesus. I still remember part of
the lyrics: *". . . O what peace we often forfeit, O what
needless pain we bear, All because we do not carry,
Everything to God in prayer."*

Scripture tells us that we are created in God's
likeness and image. And God, who is neither male
nor female, is Spirit. Therefore, the essence of us
– the part of us that experiences life everlasting
and knows no illness – is Spirit. And so it is that
at any given moment we can tune into our highest sense of God consciousness, visualize health,
put aside any fear of cancer, and KNOW that all
is well.

> *". . . and, lo, I am with you alway, even
> unto the end of the world".*
>
> MATTHEW 28:20

BIBLIOGRAPHY

G. Edward Griffin. *World Without Cancer.* Second Edition. Published by American Media. Westlake Village, California.

Maureen Kennedy Salaman. *Nutrition: The Cancer Answer.* Copyright 1996. Statford Publishing.

Klaschka, Franz. *Oral Enzymes – New Approach To Cancer Treatment.* Copyright 1996. Printed in Germany. ISBN 3-910075-22-3.

OSU News (Oregon State University). November 27, 2001. *Supplement Reduces Risk of Aflatoxin-Related Liver Cancer.* Article regarding the fungus sometimes found on peanuts and other grains.

Science in Africa. *Aflatoxin in Peanut Butter.* Copyright 2001, Janice Limson.

F. Batmanghelidj, M.D. *Water: The New Immune Breakthrough & Pain and Cancer*

"Wonder Drug". Global Health Solutions, Inc. A recorded tape of a guest lecture delivered March 19, 1992. www.watercure.com

Philip E. Binzel, M.D. *Alive and Well.* copyright 1994. American Media. Westlake Village, California.

World Cancer Research Fund. *Food, Nutrition and the Prevention of Cancer: A Global Perspective.* 1997. Source: Cornell Cooperative Extension, www.cce.cornell.edu/programs/food.

Eydie Mae with Chris Loeffler. *How I Conquered Cancer.* Copyright 1992. Avery (A member of Penguin Putnam).

William Donald Kelley, D.D. S., M.S. *One Answer To Cancer.* Copyright 1998. Published by College of Metabolic Medicine. Winfield, Kansas.

William Donald Kelley D.D.S., M.S;   Carol Morrison-Kelley, M.D.; and Kath P. Fairbanks, PhD. *Cancer Cure.* Copyright 2000. A pamphlet with articles. P.O. Box 195. Winfield, Kansas 67156.

John Beard, Doctor of Science. *The Enzyme Treatment of Cancer And Its Scientific Basis.* Copyright 1911. London, Chatto & Windus. These include copies of the originally collected papers dealing with the origin, nature, and scientific treatment of the natural phenomenon known as malignant disease.

Dr. Edward Howell. *Enzyme Nutrition.* Copyright 1985. Avery, a member of Penguin Putnam, Inc. ISBN 0-89529-221-1. Dr. Howell was born in 1898, and as of 1985 was still alive and leading an active life. He passed the board examination as a medical doctor in Illinois. A pioneer in the field of enzymes, he first wrote *The Status of Food Enzymes in Digestion and Metabolism* in 1946. He then took 20 years to complete *Enzyme Nutrition.*

Ernst T. Krebs, Jr., Ernst T. Krebs Sr. and Howard H. Beard *The Unitarian or Trophoblastic Thesis of Cancer*, as printed in the *Medical Record*, 163:149-174, July 1950.

Dr. Patrick Quillin. *Beating Cancer With Nutrition.* Copyright 1994. The Nutrition Times Press, Inc. Tulsa, Oklahoma.

Stephen R. Krauss. *O₂xygen: Nature's Most Important Dietary Supplement.* Copyright 1999. BIO2 Publishing Company. San Luis Obispo, CA 93405.

June de Spain. *The Little Cyanide Cookbook: Delicious Recipes Rich in Vitamin B17.* Get this book at your local library and if necessary, request it through inter-library loan.

Phillip Day. *Cancer: Why We're Still Dying to Know the Truth.* Credence Publications. United Kingdom. Third Edition, January 2001. ISBN 0953501238. See www.credence.org. This book is a must read if you want to get an idea of the politics of cancer.

INDEX

OTHER BOOKS BY MAURIS L. EMEKA

Heart and Soul of The Train – Personal travel notes from an Amtrak attendant. Copyright 1999. The author shares his experiences of having worked on-board Amtrak trains for more than ten years. Extracted largely from Mr. Emeka's personal travel journal, Heart and Soul of The Train takes the reader into the world of passenger train travel through interesting anecdotes and experiences on the rails. It ends with valuable travel tips for the uninitiated train traveler.

AMTRAKing – A Guide to Enjoyable Train Travel. Copyright 1994. It is clear from reading this 116-page paperback that it is written by an experienced train employee, Mauris Emeka. It addresses exactly what a person needs to know to enjoy long distance train travel in the USA. Here is a train travel guide written from an insider's point of view. It also contains an interesting chapter on the history of passenger rail travel in the USA.

Black Banks, Past And Present, copyright 1970, is a history of Black-owned commercial banks between 1865 to 1970. This book begins with an in depth look at the Freedmen's Bank which served newly freed African slaves, and it examines the operations of subsequent Black-owned banks in the USA through 1970. This book is adapted from Mr. Emeka's master's theses which he wrote as a requirement for receiving the MBA degree from the University of Washington in 1970.

To order: copy the order form at right and mail it, or notify us via E-mail

Apollo Publishing International
P.O. Box 1937
Port Orchard, Washington 98366
E-mail: emekam@silverlink.net

The author is donating a
portion of the proceeds from the sale
of Fear Cancer No More
to the Cancer Cure Foundation,
a non-profit organization in
Newbury Park, California,
whose website is: www.cancure.org

ORDER FORM

Date: _____

☐ Send me _____ copies of the book **Fear Cancer No More**, copyright 2002, at $11.95 per copy and $3 for postage and handling. Reference ISBN 0-9640125-6-1.

☐ Send me _____ copies of the book **Heart and Soul of The Train**, copyright 1999, at $9.95 per copy, and $3 for postage and handling. Reference, ISBN 0-9640125-5-3.

☐ Send me _____ copies of the book **AMTRAKing**, copyright 1994, at $8.95 per copy, and $3 for postage and handling. Reference, ISBN 0-9640125-0-2.

☐ Send me _____ copies of the book **Black Banks, Past And Present**, copyright 1970 at $15 per copy, and $3 postage and handling.

Your Name _____

Address _____

City _____ State _____ Zip _____

E-mail (optional): _____

Enclosed is a check or money order in the amount of $_____ made out to: Apollo Publishing.

To pay using Visa or MasterCard, print your name above as shown on the card, and list the card number and expiration date on the lines below:

Card #_____ Exp. Date: _____

Name as Shown on Card _____

Amount to be charged: $_____

Your signature authorization: _____